Toxins of Animal and Plant Origin

Volume 2

International Symposium on Animal and Plant
Toxins, 2d, Tel-Aviv, 1970.

Toxins of Animal and Plant Origin

Volume 2

Edited by
A. de VRIES and E. KOCHVA
Tel-Aviv University, Tel-Aviv, Israel

GORDON AND BREACH SCIENCE PUBLISHERS
New York   London   Paris

Proceedings of the Second International Symposium on Animal and Plant Toxins, held at Tel-Aviv University, Tel-Aviv, Israel, February 22–28, 1970.

PREFACE

The field of research of toxins from various sources, mainly animal, has been active during the last two decades and has resulted in several international meetings, and in a series of original and review publications. There has been rapid progress in this field, not only in its clinical and pharmacological aspects, but also on the cellular and molecular level. The knowledge accumulating is so extensive and intensive that it is imperative from time to time to review together the activities of the numerous laboratories occupied with toxin research throughout the world. Such a survey of the field was made possible by the Second International Symposium on Animal and Plant Toxins held at Tel-Aviv University in February 1970, the proceedings of which are presented here. The participants of the Symposium have covered in their papers not only the results of accomplished studies, but also preliminary findings obtained in their laboratories.

We have included in these volumes both extensive reviews and original technical reports, arranged according to disciplines rather than taxonomy. We have restricted editing to the bare minimum necessary for better comprehension and organisation of the material.

In these tasks we were aided by several colleagues from Tel-Aviv University who read some of the manuscripts, especially Drs. A. Ar, A. Bdolah, S. Ben-Efraim and B. Moaz. Mrs. Ruth Manneberg, the secretary of the Department of Zoology, Tel-Aviv University, took charge of the arranging of the manuscripts and the preparation of the book for the printer and Miss Ziva Yehezkel compiled the subject index. We thank them all for their efforts, and Gordon and Breach of London and their local representative, Miss Miriam Balaban for dealing so patiently and efficiently with the extensive texts and numerous illustrations.

A. de VRIES and E. KOCHVA

Tel-Aviv

DEDICATION

The Proceedings of the Second International Symposium on Animal and Plant Toxins, Tel-Aviv, February 1970, are dedicated to the memory of three distinguished toxinologists – Prof. O. G. Cesaire from Dakar, Senegal; Dr. Brisbois from Brussels, Belgium; and Dr. Lauhatirananda from Bangkok, Thailand. All three perished on their way to the Symposium, in the airplane that exploded over Switzerland.

They were humane, brilliant scientists. May their example serve to raise the moral status of mankind, in whose service they died.

Olivier Georges Cesaire

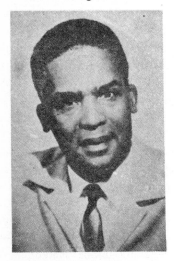

Le Professeur Olivier Georges Cesaire, né le 28 mai 1921 à Basse-Pointe, département de la Martinique, a trouvé la mort tragiquement le 21 février 1970 en se rendant à Tel-Aviv pour représenter parmi nous l'Université de Dakar.

Après de brillantes études secondaires faites à Paris, le Professeur Cesaire s'oriente vers la Pharmacie, mais ses études seront interrompues par la deuxième guerre mondiale. Il y participe depuis Alger et sert en qualité de pharmacien auxiliaire pendant les campagnes d'Italie, puis de France de 1942 à 1945. Après la libération il termine en 1946 son diplôme d'Etat de Pharmacien, puis poursuit ses études scientifiques en préparant une licence ès sciences et en soutenant sa thèse de doctorat d'état à Alger en 1950.

Chef de Travaux de Chimie Biologique à Alger de 1947 à 1955, il est ensuite détaché dans un poste équivalent à Dakar. En 1959, il est chargé des fonctions de Maître de Conférences de Chimie Analytique, puis agrégé des Facultés de Médecine et Pharmacie au concours de 1961.

En 1967, il est nommé Professeur titulaire de la chaire de Chimie Analytique et Toxicologie à la Faculté de Médecine et de Pharmacie de Dakar.

Titulaire de nombreuses distinctions honorifiques, Françaises et Sénégalaises, il était membre de sociétés savantes de réputation internationale.

Très tôt il devait orienter ses recherches vers l'analyse biologique, domaine dans lequel il rédigea plus de cinquante publications.

Homme de science certes, mais homme de coeur aussi, il était attentif à tout problème humain qu'il excellait à résoudre avec clarté et modestie. Il laisse dans sa famille, parma ses collaborateurs, ses confrères, ses amis et ses étudiants, un vide profond.

Léopold Brisbois

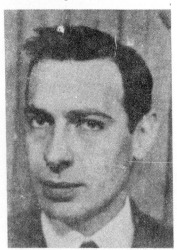

Léopold Brisbois was among the victims of the explosion of the Swissair 'Coronado' that occurred Saturday, February 21, 1970 at Wuerellingen (Switzerland). Born at Schaerbeek on June 1, 1939, married and father of a four year old child, he lived at Dilbeek. In 1962, Mr. Brisbois obtained with distinction the title of technical Engineer of Chemical Industries at the 'Institut des Industries de Fermentation – Institut Meurice Chimie'. After being employed for several months as a research worker at the 'Centre de Recherche des Substances Naturelles' he entered the O.C.D. service as a teacher in a college at Bujumbura. During his stay in Africa he took the examinations required to obtain the certificate of biochemistry at the University of Bujumbura. When he came back to Belgium he worked at 'CPRS – CERIA'. In 1966 he obtained the title of technical Engineer of Chemical Industries and Sciences with the greatest distinction. He presented two works entitled 'Contribution à l'étude des venins d'ophidiens, filtration avec gel moléculaire' and 'Etude analytique des éléments rencontrés dans les venins de serpents'. He planned to present his doctoral thesis at the University of Lille (France) in March, 1970.

Mr. Brisbois devoted his research work to snake venoms and particularly to the Formosan cobra venom

(*Naja naja atra*). He was interested not only in the biochemical aspect (purification of fractions and structural determination) but also in physiology (attenuation of pain and inhibition of malignant cells).

Mr. Brisbois will leave all his colleagues in teaching and research the memory of an intelligent, persevering and courteous man.

Dr. Prasit Lauhatirananda

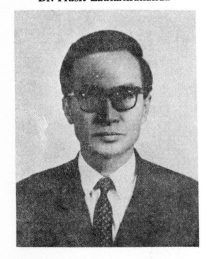

Dr. Prasit Lauhatirananda was born on 15 May 1924 in Prae, a northern province of Thailand. He obtained his medical degree from Siriraj Faculty of Medicine, University of Medical Sciences, in 1946. Immediately after graduation he joined the staff of the Queen Saovabha Memorial Institute, Thai Red Cross Society. His entire professional career was spent at this Institute where he served practically in all sections, namely, Serum Section, Vaccine Section and Research Section. His last appointment was Chief of Research Section from 1964 to the time of his death.

Dr. Lauhatirananda went abroad on several occasions for training: (1) in BCG vaccine production at the State Serum Institute, Copenhagen, (2) in vaccine and serum production at Istituto Superiore di Sanita, Rome and (3) in biological standardization at the World Health Organization Laboratory, State Serum Institute, Copenhagen. In 1963 he headed a team to demonstrate the extraction of venoms from Thailand poisonous snakes at the International Red Cross Centenary Celebration in Geneva.

After his return from training in biological standardization in Copenhagen, he took charge of the assays of cobra venom and antivenin in collaboration with the World Health Organization. He was the active investigator in the research studies on the effects of radiation on cobra venom, working in collaboration with the Office of Atomic Energy for Peace in Bangkok under a contract with the International Atomic Energy Agency in Vienna. In this connection he participated in both panel meetings arranged by the International Atomic Energy Agency in Bangkok in 1968 and 1969.

Dr. Lauhatirananda met his tragic death on 21 February 1970 in the airplane explosion in Zurich on his journey to Tel-Aviv to attend the Second International Symposium on Animal and Plant Toxins. He is survived by his wife, a seven-year-old daughter and a six-year-old son.

Volume 2

Volume 1

I GENERAL

Papers I-1 to I-5

II VENOM GLANDS AND SECRETION

Papers II-1 to II-8

III BIOCHEMISTRY (Snakes)

Papers III-1 to III-19

Volume 3

V IMMUNOLOGY

Papers V-1 to V-11

VI CLINICAL ASPECTS

Papers VI-1 to VI-11

Subject Index

BIOCHEMISTRY (OTHER SPECIES)

PROTEOLYTIC ACTIVITY OF A SPIDER VENOM

D. MEBS

Institut für Rechtsmedizin der Universität Frankfurt a.M., Germany

IN ONE OF THE FEW investigations dealing with enzymes in spider venoms Kaiser (1953) was able to demonstrate proteolytic activity in the venoms of *Ctenus nigriventer* and *Lycosa raptoria*. Recently we had the opportunity to study the proteolytic properties of a tarantula venom, *Pamphobeteus roseus*, Mello-Leitao, 1923 (Orthognatha, family: Dipluridae), kindly supplied by Prof. Bücherl, Instituto Butantan, Sao Paulo, Brazil.

Tested on casein hydrolysis (Kunitz, 1947, one unit of enzyme activity was defined as the amount of enzyme, which caused an increase of absorbancy of 0.001 at 280 nm after 20 minutes incubation at 37 °C) the crude venom showed a specific activity, 8,250 U/mg, comparable to that of snake venoms of *Crotalus* or *Bothrops* species (*Bothrops nummifera* 8,700 U/mg, *Crotalus atrox* 7,200 U/mg. Mebs, [1970].

By several steps of gel filtration (Figure 1), at first of the crude venom on Sephadex G-50, then of the proteolytic active fractions on Sephadex G-75, G-50 and Biogel P-60, three fractions were obtained called A, B, and C, showing the following properties: Their pH-optimum of casein hydrolysis is located around pH 8.5 (Figure 2). Whereas casein is digested in high rate of hydrolysis by all three protease fractions (A = 17,500 U/mg, B = 25,000 U/mg, C = 15,600 U/mg), neither the amino acid esters N-benzoyl-L-arginine ethylester (BAEE), p-toluenesulphonyl-L-arginine methylester (TAME),– both esters are substrates for trypsin–, nor N-acetyl-L-tyrosine ethylester (ATEE),–a chymotrypsin substrate–, nor N-benzoyl-DL-arginine-p-nitroanilide (BAPA) are affected. The enzyme fractions are not inhibited by Trasylol (100 IU), soybean or ovomucoid inhibitor (50 μg each, preincubated

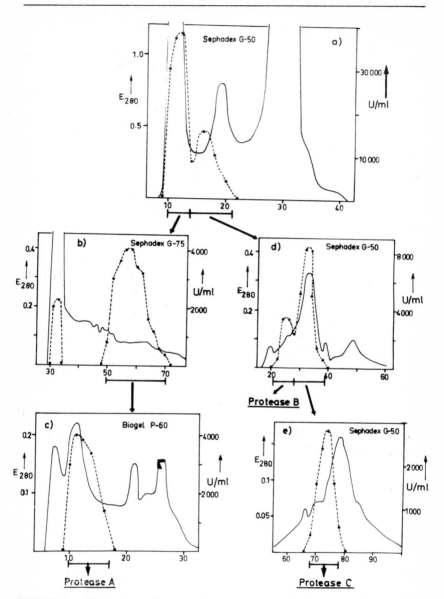

FIGURE 1.   Chromatographic separation of protease activity of *Pamphobeteus roseus* venom
a) Gel filtration of 52 mg crude venom on a Sephadex G-50 column (0.9 × 90 cm), eluted with 0.06 M phosphate buffer pH 7.0 (2 ml fractions); proteolytic activity (broken line) tested on casein hydrolysis was expressed in units (U) per ml. b) Chromatography of the first proteolytic active fraction on Sephadex G-75 (1.5 × 130 cm column, 2 ml fractions) and c) on Biogel P-60 (100–200 mesh, 1.1 × 58 cm column, 2 ml fractions, 0.06 M phosphate buffer pH 7.0). d) and e) Rechromatography of the second proteolytic active fraction on Sephadex G-50 (d) 1.5 × 70 cm column and e) 1.5 × 150 cm column, 2 ml fractions)

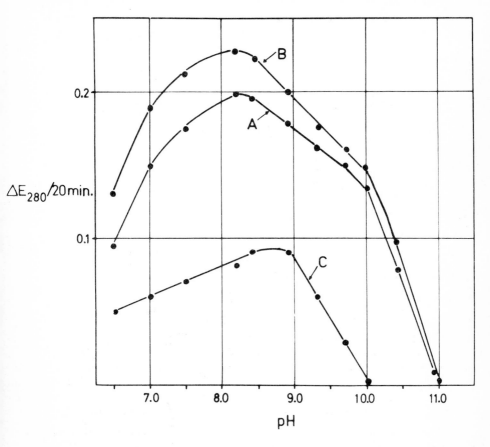

FIGURE 2.   pH-optimum of the three protease fractions, tested on casein hydrolysis in
the buffer system 0.04 M phosphoric acid, acetic acid and boric acid; the pH-value was
titrated with 0.2 N NaOH

with 5–10 μg enzyme for 60 minutes at 37 °C, pH 7.5). Likewise the trypsin
specific inhibitor N-tosyl-L-lysyl-chloromethane (5 mM) and the chymotrypsin specific inhibitor N-tosyl-L-phenylalanyl-chloromethane (5 mM) have no
effect on the enzyme activity.

The molecular weight was estimated by thin-layer-gel chromatography on

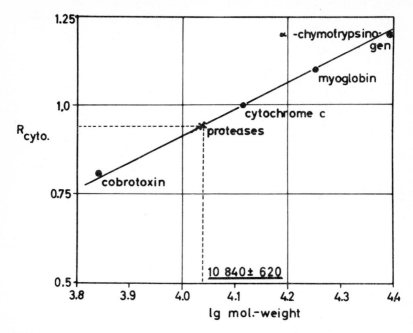

FIGURE 3.   Molecular weight determination of the protease fractions by thin-layer-gel chromatography on Sephadex G-50 (superfine) using 0.05 M tris-HC1-buffer pH 8.0 + 0.5 M NaC1 as eluent

Sephadex G-50 (superfine) using cobrotoxin (mol.w. 6,950 [Yang *et al.*, 1969]), cytochrome c (mol.w. 13,000), myoglobin (mol.w. 17,800) and α-chymotrypsinogen (mol.w. 25,000) as standard compounds (Figure 3). The protease fractions showed the same diffusion velocity refered to that of cytochrome c ($R_{cyto.}$). A molecular weight of 10,840 ± 620 was calculated.

Since all three proteases possess the same enzymatic properties and the same molecular weight, one could assume that it might probably be the same protease, which was split by gel filtration into three fractions as a result of aggregating to oligomeric forms or of complex formation.

Proteases of similarly low molecular weight were detected only in invertebrates (Arthropoda). Sonneborn *et al.* (1969) purified a protease with a molecular weight of 12,500 from the mid gut of the hornet larva (*Vespa orientalis*), possessing chymotryptic properties. A protease with a molecular weight of 11,000 and similar enzymatic properties like the spider venom proteases was isolated by Pfleiderer *et al.* (1967) from the crayfish *Astacus fluviatilis.* The high proteolytic activity of the spider venom indicates its significance for the extracorporal digestion. Furthermore, low molecular weight proteases are of great interest in the elucidation of the evolution of endopeptidases.

References

Kaiser. E. 1953 'The enzymatic activity of spider venom.' *Mem. Inst. Butantan.* **25**: 35.

Kunitz, M. 1947 'Crystalline soybean trypsin inhibitor.' *J. Gen. Physiol.*, 30: 291.

Mebs, D. 1970 'A comparative study of enzyme activities in snake venoms.' *Intern. J. Biochem.* **1**: 335.

Pfleiderer, G., R. Zwilling and H. H. Sonneborn 1967 'Eine Protease vom Molekulargewicht 11,000 und eine trypsinähnliche Fraktion aus *Astacus fluviatilis* Fabr.' *Hoppe-Seyler's Z. Physiol. Chem.*, 348: 1319.

Sonneborn, H. H., G. Pfleiderer and J. Ishay 1969 'Eine Protease vom Molekulargewicht 12,500 aus Larven von *Vespa orientalis* F. mit chymotryptischen Eigenschaften.' *Hoppe-Seyler's Z. Physiol. Chem.*, **350**: 389.

Yang, C. C., C. C. Chang, K. Hayashi and I. Suzuki 1969 'Amino acid composition and end group analysis of cobrotoxin.' *Toxicon*, 7: 43.

BIOCHEMISTRY OF *HELODERMA* VENOM

D. MEBS

Institut für Rechtsmedizin der Universität Frankfurt a.M., West Germany

INTRODUCTION

THERE IS only one venomous lizard family among the reptiles, the Gila monsters (Helodermatidae), with two species: the North American *Heloderma suspectum* (Figure 1) and the Mexican *Heloderma horridum*. Their venom glands are located in the lower jaw and as we were able to show in earlier investigations (Mebs and Raudonat, 1966, 1967; Mebs, 1968, 1969a), they produce a venom, which possesses in addition to toxic also enzymatic properties: it contains phospholipase A, hyaluronidase, esterolytic- and kinin-releasing activities.

In the following paper the fractionation of the venom of *Heloderma suspectum* and the isolation and properties of an arginine ester hydrolyzing and of a kinin-releasing enzyme (kallikrein) from this venom are reported.

MATERIALS AND METHODS

Lyophilized venom of *Heloderma suspectum* was purchased from Miami Serpentarium, Miami, USA. The hydrolysis of N-benzoyl-L-arginine ethylester (BAEE) and of p-toluene-sulphonyl-L-arginine methylester (TAME) was assayed according to the spectrophotometric method of Schwert and Takenaka (1955), the hydrolysis of N-benzoyl-DL-arginine-p-nitroanilide (BAPA) was assayed colorimetrically according to Erlanger *et al.* (1961). Casein hydrolysis was tested according to Kunitz method (1947), one unit was defined as the amount of enzyme which caused an increase of absorbancy of 0.001 at 280 nm after 20 minutes incubation at 37° C. Kinin-releasing

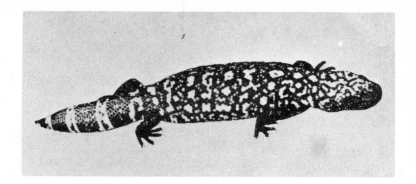

FIGURE 1.   Adult specimen of the Gila monster, *Heloderma suspectum*

activity was determined on the isolated guinea pig ileum-preparation (in aerated Tyrode-solution containing 1 mg atropine and 0.1 mg Avil per liter, at 37° C) using a 3% globulin solution (bovine plasma globulins, precipitated with ammonium sulfate between 0.3 and 0.5 fold saturation) as substrate and synthetic bradykinin (Sandoz AG, Basel, Switzerland) as standard. Specific activity was expressed in μg of synthetic bradykinin equivalents released per minute per mg enzyme.

RESULTS AND DISCUSSION

Venom fractionation by column chromatography

400 mg of crude *Heloderma* venom, dissolved in 3 ml 0.05 M sodium acetate-buffer pH 7.0 was first filtrated on a Sephadex G-75 column (Figure 2). Two BAEE-hydrolyzing fractions were obtained, of which the first one contained the kinin-releasing activity, but not the second one which was more active in arginine ester hydrolysis and still had toxic properties. For the purification of the kinin-releasing enzyme, the kallikrein fraction I desalted on a Sephadex G-25 column was applied onto a DEAE-cellulose column and eluted with a linear gradient of increasing buffer concentration (0.005 M to 0.5 M acetate buffer pH 7.0). Under these conditions (Figure 3) most of the adsorbed protein remained irreversibly bound to the cellulose and the BAEE-hydrolyzing and kinin-releasing fraction was obtained free of phospholipase A activity. The rechroma-

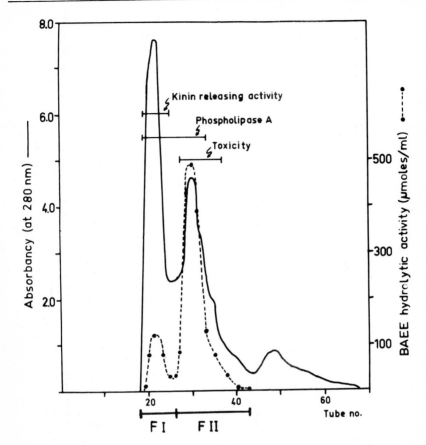

FIGURE 2.   Gel filtration of 400 mg crude venom of *Heloderma suspectum* on Sephadex G-75 (1.5 × 140 cm column), eluted with 0.05 M acetate buffer pH 7.0. The fractions (5 ml) containing kallikrein (F I, kinin-releasing and arginine ester hydrolytic) and arginine esterase activity (F II) were lyophilized and desalted on a Sephadex G-25 column (2.2 × 80 cm)

tography of the desalted fraction on DEAE-cellulose showed a symmetrical peak. The enzyme was obtained with an 11 fold increase in its kinin-releasing activity; its esterolytic activity was about 20% of that of the crude venom.

For the purification of the arginine esterase, fraction II of the gel filtrated crude venom was chromatographed on DEAE-cellulose (Figure 4). By stepwise elution with increasing buffer concentrations (sodium acetate

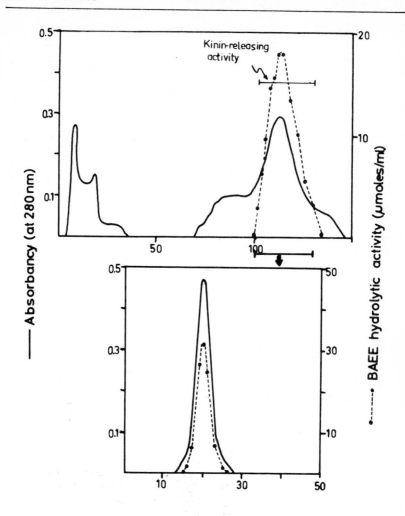

FIGURE 3.   Purification of the kallikrein of *Heloderma* venom. Above: fraction I of the Sephadex G-75 column was applied onto a DEAE-cellulose-column (2.2 × 15 cm, DEAE-SN, 0.40–0.54 meq./g, from SERVA, Heidelberg, Germany) and eluted with a linear gradient of 0.005–0.5 M acetate buffer pH 7.0. The fractions (2.5 ml) containing kinin-releasing and BAEE-hydrolyzing activity were combined, lyophilized and desalted on Sephadex G-25

Below: rechromatography of the kallikrein fraction on DEAE-cellulose (1 × 12 cm column) by gradient elution with 0.1–1.0 M acetate buffer pH 7.0 (4.5 ml fractions)

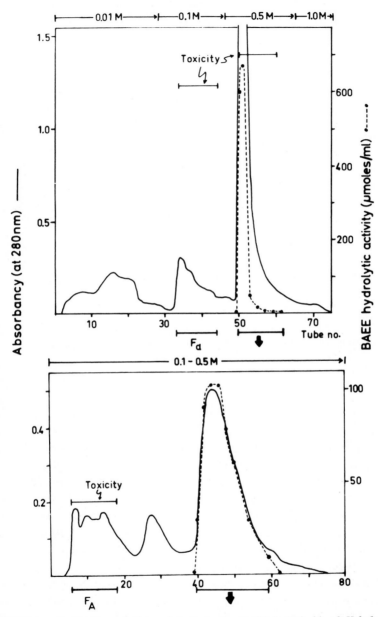

FIGURE 4.   Purification of the arginine esterase (BAEE-hydrolysis) of *Heloderma* venom. Above: fraction II of the Sephadex G-75 column (figure 2) was applied onto a DEAE-cellulose-column (1.5 × 12 cm), stepwise elution was carried out starting with 0.01 M acetate buffer pH 7.0 and increasing the buffer concentration until 1.0 M. The enzyme fraction, lyophilized and desalted on Sephadex G-25, was chromatographed on a DEAE-cellulose column (1.5 × 7 cm, below) using linear gradient elution (0.1–0.5 M acetate buffer pH 7.0)

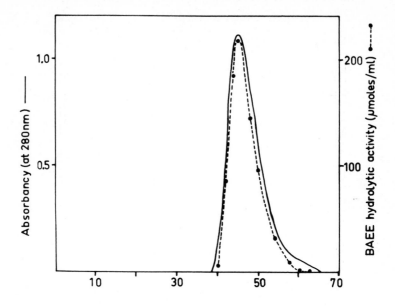

FIGURE 5.   Gel filtration of the arginine esterase fraction (figure 3) on Biogel P-60 (100–200 mesh, 1.5 × 150 cm), eluted with 0.05 M acetate buffer pH 7.0

buffer pH 7.0) three fractions were obtained, of which the second one (F_a) possessed toxic properties; however, the arginine esterase fraction still remained toxic. From this latter fraction, a further toxic fraction (F_A) was separated by rechromatography on DEAE-cellulose using a linear buffer gradient (0.1 to 0.5 M acetate buffer pH 7.0). Gel filtration of the arginine esterase fraction on Biogel P-60 gave a symmetrical peak (Figure 5). The enzyme was obtained 8.5 fold enriched, its BAEE-hydrolyzing activity was about 80 per cent of the crude venom activity.

The two toxic fractions, separated in the course of purifying the arginine esterase, were filtrated on a Sephadex G-75 column exactly under the same conditions. In the elution pattern (Figure 6), both fractions show a corresponding position of their toxic peaks, suggesting that we might probably deal with the same toxin, which was incompletely separated from

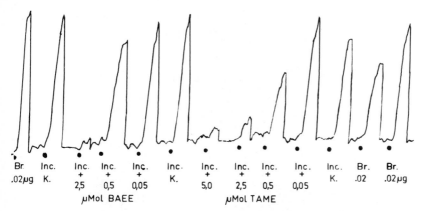

FIGURE 8.   Inhibition of kinin-releasing activity of *Heloderma*-kallikrein by BAEE and TAME, tested on the isolated guinea pig ileum. Br. = synthetic bradykinin per 10 ml Tyrode-bath; Inc. = 0.02 ml of the reaction mixture consisting of 5 μg enzyme (0.05 ml) preincubated for one minute with BAEE or TAME at 37° C, and 0.5 ml 3% plasma-globulin solution as substrate (3 min incubation at 37° C); K = control reaction mixture without BAEE or TAME

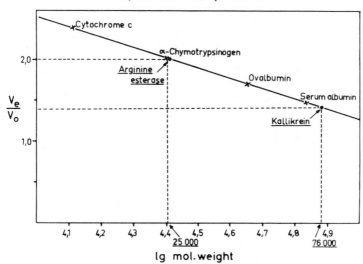

FIGURE 9.   Molecular weight determination of kallikrein and arginine esterase by gel filtration on Sephadex G-100 (1.5 × 100 cm column, 0.05 M tris-HCl-buffer pH 7.3 + 0.5 M NaCl). V_e = elution volume; V_o = void volume

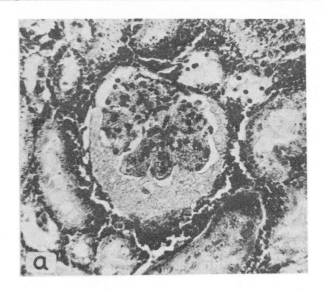

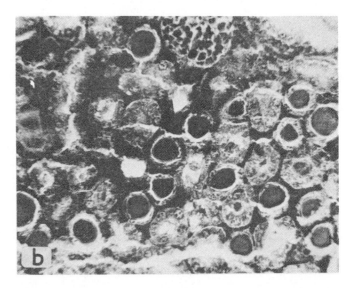

FIGURE 10.   Histological sections of the kidney and the eyeball of a mouse (20 g)
24 hrs after s.c. injection of 35 μg arginine esterase fraction. Goldner's trichrome:
a) kidney; the space of Bowman's capsule filled with a fibrous, granular substance,
     400 x,
b) kidney; tubules with hyaline cylinders in the lumen, 250 x,

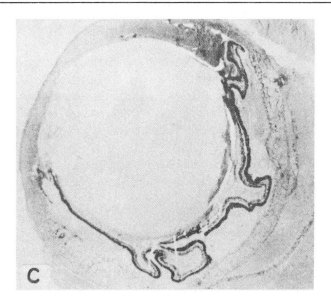

c) eyeball showing retinal detachment by haemorrhages, 25 x

During the toxicity tests of the crude venom on mice it was observed, that those animals surviving several hours showed exophthalmus and massive haemorrhages of the eye ball. Similar observations had been made by Kornalik (personal communication) with *Heloderma* venom. The fractionation of the venom revealed that this haemorrhagic effect is obviously due to the arginine esterase fraction. However, this enzyme fraction itself has a lethal effect only in relatively high doses (6–7 μg/g mouse). The examination of the animals reveals large haemorrhages of the intestines, swollen kidneys and occasionally bleedings in the lungs. With lower doses (1–2 μg/g mouse) the animals survived 2–3 days or longer. In most of this cases the kidneys are damaged by massive haemorrhages. The microscopic examination yields the following findings (Figure 10): the kidney is enlarged by interstitial haemorrhages around the tubules and Bowman's capsules. Tubular necrosis is also seen affecting the distal as well as the proximal convoluted tubules. The lumina of the tubules and the space of Bowman's capsules are filled with a granular or hyaline substance. Usually both kidneys are affected, thus renal failure may be the cause of the death in animals, which died after two or three days. Around the eyeball the connective tissue is interspersed with massive haemorrhages producing the observed exophthalmus. Mostly retinal detachment occurs after bleeding into the eyebulb.

If the arginine esterase is inhibited by DFP, the inactive enzyme separated from the remaining DFP by gel filtration on Sephadex G-25, shows the same pathological changes in mice after subcutaneous injection. Thus an enzymatic effect due to the arginine esterase can be excluded, suggesting that the enzyme fraction still contains a factor with haemorrhagic properties.

While one of the arginine ester hydrolyzing enzymes in the venom of *Heloderma suspectum* was defined as kallikrein, because of its kinin-releasing activity, further characterization of the second enzyme was not achieved, as its natural substrate and physiological significance is still unknown. However, it could be confirmed, that this enzyme is involved neither in the toxic nor in the haemorrhagic effects of the venom.

SUMMARY

The venom of the only poisonous lizard *Heloderma suspectum* was fractionated by gel filtration and column chromatography on DEAE-cellulose. Two enzymes active in hydrolyzing arginine esters (N-benzoyl-L-arginine ethylester and p-toluene-sulphonyl-L-arginine ethylester) were isolated, of which one was characterized as kallikrein, releasing kinin from plasma globulins. The other arginine esterase could be separated from the toxic principle of the venom, but was still contaminated with a factor which causes massive haemorrhages predominantly of the kidneys and eyes of mice.

References

Cohen, I., M. Zur, E. Kaminsky and A. de Vries 1969 'Isolation and characterization of kinin-releasing enzyme of *Echis coloratus* venom.' *Toxicon*, 7: 3.

Erlanger, B. F., N. Kokowsky and W. Cohen 1961 'The preparation and properties of two new chromogenic substrates of trypsin.' *Arch. Biochem. Biophys.*, 95: 271.

Frey, E. K., H. Kraut and E. Werle 1968 *'Das Kallikrein-Kinin-System und seine Inhibitoren.'* Ferdinand Enke Verlag, Stuttgart.

Iwanaga, S., T. Sato, Y. Mizushima and T. Suzuki 1965 'Studies on snake venoms. XVII. Properties of the bradykinin releasing enzyme in the venom of *Agkistrodon halys blomhoffii.*' *J. Biochem. (Tokyo)*, 58: 123.

Kunitz, M. 1947 'Crystalline soybean trypsin inhibitor.' *J. Gen. Physiol.*, 30: 291.

Mebs, D. 1968 'Some studies on the biochemistry of the venom gland of *Heloderma horridum.' Toxicon*, **5**: 225.

Mebs, D. 1969a 'Isolierung und Eigenschaften eines Kallikreins aus dem Gift der Krustenechse *Heloderma suspectum.' Hoppe-Seyler's Z. physiol. Chem.*, 350: 821.

Mebs, D. 1969b 'Über Schlangengift-Kallikreine: Reinigung und Eigenschaften eines kininfreisetzenden Enzyms aus dem Gift der Viper *Bitis gabonica.' Hoppe-Seyler's Z. Physiol. Chem.*, **350**: 1563.

Mebs, D. and H. W. Raudonat 1966 'Biochemical investigations on *Heloderma* venom.' *Mem. Inst. Butantan*, **33**: 907.

Mebs, D. and H. W. Raudonat, 1967 'Biochemie des Giftes der Krustenechsen *Heloderma suspectum* und *Heloderma horridum.' Naturwissenschaften*, **54**: 494.

Schwert, G. W. and Y. Takenaka 1955 'A spectrophotometric determination of trypsin and chymotrypsin.' *Biochim. Biophys. Acta*, **16**: 570.

Werle, E. and B. Kaufmann-Boetsch 1959 'Über eine esterspaltende Wirkung von Kallikrein.' *Naturwissenschaften*, **46**: 559.

Whitaker, J. R. 1963 'Determination of molecular weights of proteins by gel filtration on Sephadex.' *Anal. Chem.*, **35**: 1950.

ON THE TOXIN OF EUROPEAN
BOMBINA SPECIES

A. CSORDAS and H. MICHL

Department of Chemistry, University of Agriculture, Vienna, Austria

INTRODUCTION

THE SKIN SECRETION of European *Bombina* species contains proteins, peptides, amino acids and 5-hydroxytryptamine (Kiss and Michl, 1962). Some of these substances show biological activities, e.g. cytotoxic and antibiotic action of some proteins and peptides (Kaiser *et al.*, 1964; Bachmayer *et al.*, 1967) and inflammation produced by 5-hydroxytryptamine (Garattini and Valzelli, 1965). These components cause defensive effects of skin secretion against predators and microorganisms. Of all these substances a hemolytic and surface active tetracosane peptide ('bombinin') deserves special consideration (Csordas and Michl, 1969, 1970). Immediately after milking the skin secretion contains a fair percentage (1–10%) of it. After an hour at room temperature, however, most of it is hydrolysed by enzymes of the toxin causing a considerable loss of the heat stable hemolytic activity. At the same time an increase of the concentration of the peptides 2, 4 and probably 7 takes place (Molzer, 1970). This process may offer some protection against self poisoning of the animals.

MATERIAL AND METHODS

Toxin

The milking procedure is done as previously described (Kiss and Michl, 1962). The toxin is deep-frozen immediately after its preparation and freeze-dried as quickly as possible.

Purification of bombinin

		Recovery
Step 1:	*Fractionated precipitation with acetone*	*20 mg(5%)*
	400 mg freeze-dried toxin are dissolved in 30 ml pyridine-acetate buffer pH 4.7 (10 ml pyridine, 10 ml glacial acetic acid per liter). 90 ml cold ($-20°$) acetone is added. The white precipitate is spun down in a refrigerated centrifuge and discarded. The supernatant fluid is diluted with the same volume of cold acetone and centrifuged.	amino-acids, bombinin, peptides 4, 4a and 5
Step 2:	*Sephadex filtration*	*12 mg(3%)*
	20 mg of the precipitate are dissolved in 3 ml dist. water and placed on a 1.5 cm diameter column containing 120 ml Sephadex G-25. The column is eluted with dist. water. The bombinin containing fractions are pooled and freeze-dried.	peptides 4, 4a and 5, bombinin
Step 3:	*Thin layer chromatography*	*7 mg(1,8%)*
	The coating material is powdered cellulose MN 30 (Macherey-Nagel, Durel, Germany), the developing solvent a mixture of n-propanol: pyridine-acetate buffer pH 4.7 in ratio 2:1 (v/v). The R_F-value of bombinin is 0.78	bombinin, some peptides
Step 4:	*High voltage paper electrophoresis at pH 4.7*	*4 mg(1%)*
	Whatman 3 MM papers and pyridine-acetate buffer are used.	bombinin
Step 5:	*High voltage paper electrophoresis at pH 2.0*	*2 mg(0,5%)*
	Whatman 3 MM papers and a buffer containing 25 ml formic acid (80%) and 87 ml glacial acetic acid per liter are used.	bombinin

Enzymatic degradation

Degradation is made with chymotrypsin (Fluka A 52342) and trypsin (Fluka A 58123). The hydrolysis is performed in acetate-ammonia buffer at pH 7.5–8.5. One ml of buffer solution contains 5% of enzyme. The incubation with trypsin lasts 8 hours (code Table 1:T), with chymotrypsin 25 minutes (code: Chs) and 6 hours (code: Chl), respectively. Chromatography and high voltage electrophoresis of the degradation products, determination of the amino acid composition, and end-group analysis were accomplished according to previously described methods (Csordas and Michl, 1969, 1970).

RESULTS AND DISCUSSION

The amino acid content in molar ratios agrees with the formula Ala_6, Asp, Glu, Gly_5, His, Ile, Leu_4, Lys_3, Phe, Ser. Glycine is in the N-terminal position. The C-terminus is blocked. Bombinin contains only one aspartic acid residue. From the degradation products (Table 1) the dipeptides Chs-3 and Chl-7 contain this amino acid. They show a high cathodic migration rate which demonstrates the lack of free carboxylic groups. By comparison with previously isolated (Kiss and Michl, 1962) and synthesized (Nesvadba *et al.*, 1965) material, they were identified with $\underset{23}{Ala}-\underset{24}{Asp}(NH_2)_2$ (Table 2). Chs-3 and Chl-7 are therefore the C-terminal peptides of bombinin. The sequence of eight C-terminal amino acid residues can be deduced from hexapeptide Chl-6 and the octapeptide T-2, both containing $Ala-Asp(NH_2)_2$. Chl-6 contains the only glutaminic acid, the only histidine, and the only phenylalanine residues of bombinin. The tetrapeptide Chl-1 must be part of it. Chl-1 can be hydrolysed in the two peptides $\underset{19}{Ala}-\underset{20}{Glu}$ and $\underset{21}{His}-\underset{22}{Phe}$ again identical with previously identified dipeptides. Since the N-terminal amino acid residue of Chl-1 is alanine and the C-terminal residue is phenylalanine the sequence has to be $\underset{19}{Ala}-\underset{20}{Glu}-\underset{21}{His}-\underset{22}{Phe}$. Therefore the sequence of Chl-6 is $\underset{19}{Ala}-\underset{20}{Glu}-\underset{21}{His}-\underset{22}{Phe}-\underset{23}{Ala}-\underset{24}{Asp}(NH_2)_2$. T-2 has glycine and leucine more than Chl-6, glycine being the N-terminal residue. This proves the sequence $\underset{17}{Gly}-\underset{18}{Leu}$. The sequence down to residue 12 can be deduced mainly from the undecapeptide Chs-1 and octapeptide Chl-3 both containing the C-terminal sequence $\underset{20}{Glu}-\underset{21}{His}-\underset{22}{Phe}$. Both Chl-3 and T-2 intersect therefore from residue 17 to residue 22, Chl-3 containing the two residues alanine and lysine on the

TABLE 1   Structures of tryptic and chymotryptic peptides from Bombinin.

Code	HV-Electropho-resis at pH 4.7	Amino acid composition	N-terminal amino acid	C-terminal amino acid
T_1	0,29/Lys	$Ala_2,Gly_2,Ile,Leu,Lys,Ser$	Gly	–
T_2	0,41/Lys	$Ala_2,Asp,Glu,Gly,His,Leu,Phe$	Gly	–
T_3	0,49/Lys	Ala,Glu,Gly,His,Leu,Phe	Gly	Phe
T_4	0,64/Lys	Ala,Gly,Leu,Lys	Gly	–
Chl–0	start	Ala,Gly_2,Ile,Leu	Gly	Leu
Chl–01	start	Gly,Leu	Gly	–
Chl–1	0,13/Lys	Ala,Glu,His,Phe	Ala	Phe
Chl–2	0,37/Lys	Ala_2,Gly,Leu,Lys,Ser	Ser	Phe
Chl–3	0,41/Lys	$Ala_2,Gly,Glu,His,Leu,Lys,Phe$	Ala	–
Chl–4	0,64/Lys	Ala,Gly,Leu,Lys	Ala	Leu
Chl–5	0,69/Lys	Gly,Leu,Lys	Lys	Leu
Chl–6	0,74/Lys	Ala_2,Asp,Glu,His,Phe	Ala	–
Chl–7	0,88/Lys	Ala,Asp	Ala	–
Chs–1	0,25/Lys	$Ala_2,Gly_2,Glu,His,Leu_2,Lys_2,Phe$	Lys	–
Chs–2	0,37/Lys	Ala_2,Gly,Leu,Lys,Ser	Ser	Leu
Chs–3	0,88/Lys	Ala,Asp	Ala	–

T–Peptides after tryptic digestion for 8 hours. . .
Chl–Peptides after chymotryptic digestion for 8 hours. . .; Chs for 15 minutes. . .
Amino acids in alphabetical order.

TABLE 2   Amino acid sequence of Bombinin

```
   1   2   3   4   5   6   7   8   9  10  11  12  13  14  15  16  17  18  19  20  21  22  23  24

                                                            Ala-Lys-Gly-Leu-Ala-GluX-His-Phe
                                                                        Chl 3
                                                                                 Gly-Leu Ala-GluX-His-Phe-Ala-Asp(NH2)2
                                                                                 Chl-01        Chl-6
                                                            Gly-Leu
                                                            Chl-01
                                                   Lys-Gly-Leu Ala-Lys-Gly-Leu Ala-GluX-His-Phe
                                                   Chl-5                  Chl-4          Chl-1

Gly-Ile-Gly-Ala-Leu Ser-Ala-Lys-Gly-Ala-Leu Lys-Gly-Leu-Ala-Lys-Gly-Leu-Ala-GluX-His-Phe Ala-Asp(NH2)2
Chl-0               Chs-2,Chl-2                                                            Chs-3,Chl-7
                                                            Chs-1
                                                            Gly-Leu-Ala-GluX-His-Phe
                                                                        T-3

Gly-Ile-Gly-Ala-Leu-Ser-Ala-Lys Gly-Ala-Leu-Lys Gly-Leu-Ala-GluX-His-Phe-Ala-Asp(NH2)2
           T-1                      T-4                       T-2

Gly-Ile-Gly-Ala-Leu-Ser-Ala-Lys-Gly-Ala-Leu-Lys-Gly-Leu-Ala-Lys-Gly-Leu-Ala-GluX-His-Phe-Ala-Asp(NH2)2
                                              Bombinin
   1   2   3   4   5   6   7   8   9  10  11  12  13  14  15  16  17  18  19  20  21  22  23  24

Gly-Ile-Gly-Ala-Leu                                         Ala-Glu-His-Phe-Ala-Asp(NH2)2
   Peptide 7                                                         Peptide 2

                                 Ser -Ala-Lys-Gly-Leu-Ala-Glu  -His-Phe   Peptide 4aα
                                 Gly                                               4aβ
```

N-terminus. The tetrapeptide Chl-4 is part of Chl-3 confirming the proposed sequence. Since the N-terminal amino acid residue of Chs-1 is lysine, only the sequence of glycine and leucine in the position 13 and 14 can be deduced from the present results. The sequence Leu-Gly would be in good accordance with the previously described nonapeptides (Csordas and Michl, 1969) 4aα and 4aβ. It has been demonstrated (Molzer, 1970) that bombinin is not a precursor of the 4a-peptides. On the other hand the peptides T-4, Chl-5, and Chl-01 fit well into this part of the primary structure. Therefore the sequence Lys-Gly-Leu-Ala-Lys has been prefered.
$\quad$ 12 13 14 15 16

After hydrolysis of bombinin with trypsin four peptides (T-1, T-2, T-3, T-4,) were separated. T-2, T-3, and part of T-4 fit nicely into the sequence 13-24 just described. Thus it is supposed that T-1 is the N-terminal part of bombinin. T-1 has glycine as the N-terminal, lysine as the C-terminal amino acid, and contains the only serine and isoleucin residues of bombinin. The pentapeptide Chl-0 also contains isoleucine. The octapeptide T-1 is therefore the extension of Chl-0 containing serine, alanine, and lysine more than Chl-0. The sequence of Chl-0 is elucidated by Edman-degradation and partial hydrolysis with conc. hydrochloric acid to be Gly-Ile-Gly-Ala-Leu. Further-
$\quad$ 1   2   3   4   5
more it is probably identical with peptide 7 of the toxin (Molzer, 1970). The amino acids serine, alanine, and lysine of T-1 have to be the C-terminal sequence, lysine being the eighth amino acid residue. The identical hexa-peptides Chl-2 and Chs-2 contain N-terminal serine residues and a single lysine which must be the same as in T-1. Therefore the sequence of the N-terminus of Chl-2 and the C-terminal sequence of T-1 are Ser-Ala-Lys. The remaining
$\quad$ 6   7   8
three amino acid residues of Chs-2 and Chl-2 glycine, alanine, and leucine occupy the positions 9−11. Since leucine is the C-terminal residue it has the position 11. For the last step we have to consider the peptides T-4. Since there are three lysines in bombinin and no lys-lys-sequence, four peptides must be formed by exhaustive digestion with trypsin. One has to be free of lysine, in our case T-2 (T-3 is the result of a small chymotryptic activity of trypsin). Three peptides must contain lysine, only two peptides T-1 and T-4 have been separated. To be compatible with the gross amino acid composition of bombinin it is necessary to suggest two peptides T-4. One has the sequence Gly-Leu-Ala-Lys the other Gly-Ala-Leu-Lys. Therefore the second peptide
$\quad$ 13 14 15 16 $\qquad$ 9 10 11 12
T-4 bridges 9−12 and with it both parts of bombinin.

There is some similarity between bombinin and melittin. The sequence of the N-terminal amino acid residues 1−4 are identical (Table 3). Melittin

TABLE 3   Comparison of the primary structures of Bombinin and Melittin.

Bombinin

1	2	3	4	5	6	7	8	9	10	11	12	13	14
Gly-Ile-Gly-Ala-Leu-	Ser	-Ala-	Lys	- Gly-Ala-Leu-	Lys	-Gly-Leu-
Gly-Ile-Gly-Ala-Val -	Leu	-	Lys	- Val-Leu -	Thr-Thr	-Gly-Leu-

| 1 | 2 | 3 | 4 | 5 | 6 | 7 | 8 | 9 | 10 | 11 | 12 | 13 |

Melittin

Bombinin

15	16	17	18	19	20	21	22	23	25
Ala-	Lys	-Gly-Leu-Ala-GluX-	His	— Phe — Ala-	Asp(NH$_2$)$_2$
-Pro-Ala-Leu-Ile-	Ser	— Try — Ile-	Lys-Arg-Lys-Arg	— Glu(NH$_2$)-Glu(NH$_2$)$_2$

| 14 | 15 | 16 | 17 | 18 | 19 | 20 | 21 | 22 | 23 | 24 | 25 | 26 |

Melittin

     basic and hydrophilic amino acid residues
| identical amino acid residues

contains a lysine residue at position 7, bombinin at position 8. The basic lysine residues in position 12 and 16 of bombinin correspond with two hydrophilic threonine residues of melittin in 10 and 11 and the serine residue in 18. The accumulation of strongly basic lysine and arginine residues (21–24) of melittin is opposed only by a weekly basic histidine (21) in bombinin. The C-terminal monoaminodicarbonic acid diamides correspond well in both polypeptides. As could be expected, bombinin has a distinctly lower hemolytic activity than melittin (Molzer, 1970). A striking feature of the primary structure of bombinin is the repetition of the sequence Lys-Gly-(Ala,Leu) at the positions 8–11, 12–15, and 16–19. Similar repetitions are known to occur in fibrous proteins (Lucas and Rudall, 1968) and histones (Dayhoff, 1969). It may be mentioned that protamins and basic histones cause an agglutination of erythrocytes which resembles the first step of hemolysis by the heat stable hemolytic factor of the toxin of *Bombina*.

ACKNOWLEDGMENTS

This project is supported by 'Österreichischer Forschungsrat'. The amino acid analyzer is a gift from the 'Österreichische Nationalbank'.

SUMMARY

Some of the lower molecular peptides occuring in *Bombina* toxin are formed by splitting a higher molecular weight, melittin-like peptide into smaller fragments. This fragmentation could be avoided by deep-freezing the toxin immediately after its preparation. Subsequent separation procedures at low temperatures yielded a pure tetracosane peptide ('bombinin'). Its primary structure was investigated by known methods of protein chemistry. Similarities and dissimilarities of bombinin and melittin are discussed.

References

Bachmayer, H., H. Michl and B. Roos 1967 'Chemistry of cytotoxic substances in amphibian toxins. *In*: Russell, F. E. and P. R. Saunders (eds.) *Animal Toxins*. p. 395 Oxford: Pergamon Press.

Csordas, A. and H. Michl 1969 'Primary structure of two oligopeptides of the toxin of *Bombina variegata* L. *Toxicon*, 7: 103.

Csordas, A. and H. Michl 1970 'Isolierung und Strukturaufklärung eines hämolytisch wirkenden Polypeptides aus dem Abwehrsekret europäischer Unken. *Monatsh. Chem.*, 101: 182.

Dayhoff, M. O. 1969 '*Atlas of Protein Sequence and Structure*. National Biomedical Research Foundation, Silver Spring.

Garattini, S. and L. Valzelli 1965 '*Serotonin*.' Elsevier, Amsterdam.

Kaiser, E., H. Michl and K. Springer 1964 'Zytotoxische Wirkungen des Hautsekretes der Gelbbauchunke (*Bombina variegata* L.) *Z. Angew. Zool.*, 51: 1

Kiss, G. and H. Michl 1962 'Über das Giftsekret der Gelbbauchunke *Bombina variegata* L. *Toxicon*, 1: 33.

Lucas, F. and K. M. Rudall 1968 'Extracellular fibrous proteins, In: Florkin, M. and E. Stotz (eds.), *Comprehensive Biochemistry*. Vol. 26B p. 475. Elsevier, Amsterdam.

Molzer, H. 1970 Über Inhaltsstoffe des Abwehrsekretes europäischer Unken. Ph. D. Thesis, University of Vienna.

Nesvadba, H., H. Bachmayer and H. Michl 1965 'Über die Synthese eines im Gift von *Bombina variègata* vorkommenden Hexapeptiddiamids.' *Monatsch. Chem.*, 96: 1125

STRUCTURE OF SCORPION NEUROTOXINS

H. ROCHAT, C. ROCHAT, C. KUPEYAN, S. LISSITZKY,
F. MIRANDA and P. EDMAN

Laboratoire de Biochimie Médicale, Faculté Mixte de Médecine
et de Pharmacie, Boulevard Jean Moulin,
Marseille, France
and
St Vincent's School of Medical Research, Melbourne, Australia

---

To the memory of Professor Georges Olivier Césaire

INTRODUCTION

USING THE GENERAL METHOD of purification described in another paper (Miranda *et al.*, this volume) we have isolated 11 neurotoxins from the venoms of three different scorpions: *Androctonus australis, Buthus occitanus tunetanus* and *Leiurus quinquestriatus quinquestriatus*. In order to compare their primary structure, we determined the amino acid sequences of 4 of them: toxins I and II of *Androctonus australis*, toxin I of *Buthus occitanus tunetanus* and toxin III of *Leiurus quinquestriatus quinquestriatus*. Thus, it was possible not only to compare toxins of the same subspecies but also toxins originating from scorpions of different genera.

As these proteins are composed of a single polypetide chain cross linked by four disulfide bridges, they were submitted to the action of 2-mercaptoethanol. The cystein residues thus formed were quantitatively converted into S-methylcysteine residues (MeC) (Rochat *et al.*, 1970). Then, the methylated proteins were submitted to the Edman degradation procedure using the Protein Sequenator (Edman and Begg, 1967), and their N-terminal amino acid sequences were established.

In the case of toxin I of *Androctonus australis* the C-terminal residue was identified as threonine by hydrazinolysis (Niu and Fraenkel-Conrat, 1955).

FIGURE 1.   Aminoacid sequence of *Androctonus australis Hector* methylated Toxin I

H-Lys-Arg-Asp-Gly-Tyr-Ile-Val-Tyr-Pro-Asn-Asn-MeC-Val-Tyr-His-MeC-Val-Pro-Pro-MeC-Asp
$\qquad$ 10 $\qquad$ 20 | Gly |

Ala-Leu-Gly-Ser-Pro-Val-Leu-Phe-MeC-Ser-Ser-Gly-Ser-Ser-Gly-Gly-Asn-Lys-Lys-MeC-Leu
40 $\qquad$ 30

Try-MeC-Lys-Asp-Leu-Pro-Asp-Asn-Val-Pro-Ile-Lys-Asp-Thr-Ser-Arg-Lys-MeC-Thr-OH
50 $\qquad$ 60

MeC: S-methylcysteine

Arrows show the bonds hydrolysed by chymotrypsin

The action of carboxypeptidase A led to the following C-terminal sequence: -Lys-MeC-Thr-OH. The methylated protein was then submitted to chymotryptic hydrolysis and the 7 resulting peptides were purified by gel filtration (Sephadex G-25 and G-10) and by high voltage paper electrophoresis. The sequence of peptides was established by the Edman degradation (Blomback *et al.*, 1966), partial acidic hydrolysis and carboxypeptidase A

FIGURE 2.   Primary structure of scorpion neurotoxins

                                                     10   20
B I   H-Gly-Arg-Asp-Ala-Tyr-Ile-Ala-Gln-Pro-Glu-Asn-*MeC*-Val-Tyr-Glu-*MeC*-Ala-Gln-X – Y -*Tyr-MeC*-
L III   H-*Val*-Arg-Asp-Ala-Tyr-Ile-Ala-Lys-Asn-Tyr-Asn-*MeC*-Val-Tyr-Glu-*MeC*-Phe-Arg-Asp-Ser-*Tyr-MeC*-Asn-Asp-
A II   H-*Val*-Lys-Asp-Gly-Tyr-Ile-Val-Asp-Asp-Val-Asn-*MeC*-Thr-Tyr-Phe-*MeC*-Gly-Arg-Asn-Ala-*Tyr-MeC*-Asn-Glu-
A I   H-Lys-*Arg*-Asp-Gly-Tyr-Ile-Val-Tyr-Pro-Asn-Asn-*MeC*-Val-Tyr-His-*MeC*-Val-Pro-Pro- del. -*MeC*-Asp-Gly-
                                                                                               -Ile -
                                                                                                  20

                   30
L III   -*Leu-MeC-Thr-Lys*-
A II   -Glu-*MeC*-Thr-Lys-Leu-Lys-Gly-Glu-*Ser-Gly*-Tyr-del-*MeC*-Gln-Try-Ala-Ser-Pro-Tyr-Gly-
A I   -*Leu-MeC*-Lys-*Lys*-Asn-Gly-Gly-*Ser-Ser-MeC*-Phe-Leu-Val-Pro-Ser-Gly-Leu-Ala-MeC-Try-MeC-
                                                                 40

A I   -Lys-Asp-Leu-Pro-Asp-Asn-Val-Pro-Ile-Lys-Asp-Thr-Ser-Arg-Lys-*MeC*-Thr-OH
                                                 50   60

B I   :   Toxin I of *Buthus occitanus tunetanus*
L III :   Toxin III of *Leiurus quinquestriatus quinquestriatus*
A II :   Toxin II of *Androctonus australis Hector*
A I   :   Toxin I of *Androctonus australis Hector*

del.: deletion
MeC : S-methylcysteine

action. The results of these investigations are shown in Figure 1 which gives the primary sequence of the toxin. The heat-denaturated toxin was also submitted to the simultaneous action of both trypsin and chymotrypsin. The resulting hydrolysate was investigated by gel filtration and finger printing. Two disulfide bridges were located (between half-cystine residues 11 and 62, 24 and 46); the two others are under investigation.

Toxin I' of *Androctonus australis* is found in scorpions collected in south Tunisia. It only differs from Toxin I by the replacement of valine residue number 17 by an isoleucine residue.

Figure 2 gives the results obtained so far concerning the primary structure of scorpion neurotoxins. It can be seen that there are homologous sequences in these 4 proteins. Of particular interest is the position of the S-methylcysteine residues: if we assumed that deletions occurred in the *Androctonus australis Hector* neurotoxins, then the disulfide bridges would be in the same position in all scorpion neurotoxins.

The above results confirm that scorpion neurotoxins make up a family of proteins. Although they have common general features with the family of snake - neurotoxins, there are great differences (See Miranda *et al.*, this volume). If we compare our own results on scorpion neurotoxins with the results of others on snake neurotoxins (Botes and Strydom, 1969; Yang *et al.*, 1969; Botes, this volume; Tamiya *et al.*, this volume), it appears that the amino acid sequences are completely different. This is in a good agreement with the fact that the symptomatology of poisoning is also quite different: flaccid paralysis in the case of snakes and spastic paralysis in the case of scorpions.

References

Blombäck, B., M. Blombäck, P. Edman and B. Hessel 1966 'Human fibrinopeptides. Isolation, characterization and structure.' *Biochim. Biophys. Acta*, 115: 371–396.
Botes, D. P. and D. J. Strydom 1969 'A neurotoxin, toxin α, from Egyptian cobra (*Naja haje haje*) venom. I. Purification, properties and complete amino acid sequence. *J. Biol. Chem.*, 244: 4147–4157.
Edman, P. and G. Begg 1967 'A Protein Sequenator'. *European J. Biochem.*, 1: 80–91.
Niu, C. I. and H. Fraenkel-Conrat 1955 'Determination of C-terminal amino acids and peptides by hydrazinolysis.' *J. Amer. Chem. Soc.*, 77: 5882–5885.
Rochat, C., H. Rochat and P. Edman 1970 'Some S-alkyl derivatives of cystein suitable for sequence determination by the phenylisothiocyanate technic.' *Anal. Biochem.* 37: 259–267.
Yang, C. C., H. J. Yang and J. S. Huang 1969 'The amino acid sequence of cobrotoxin.' *Biochim. Biophys. Acta*, 188: 65–77.

PURIFICATION OF TOXINS FROM THE NORTH AMERICAN SCORPION *CENTRUROIDES SCULPTURATUS**

M. E. McINTOSH** and **D. D. WATT**†

*Department of Microbiology, Kansas University School of Medicine,
Kansas City, Kansas and Midwest Research Institute, Kansas City,
Missouri, U.S.A.*

INTRODUCTION

VENOM OF TWO North African scorpions, *Buthus occitanus* and *Androctonus australis* have been investigated and their neurotoxins purified (Miranda and Lissitzky, 1961; Miranda *et al.*, 1964a, 1964b; Rochat *et al.*, 1967; see also Rochat *et al*, this volume). The neurotoxins of the South American scorpion *Tityus serrulatus* have also been purified (Miranda *et al.*, 1966a). Venom from the three species thus far studied each contain two neurotoxins of low molecular weight.

Previous studies concerning the chemistry of the venom from the North American scorpion *Centruroides sculpturatus* have been reported (Watt, 1964; McIntosh and Watt, 1967). Watt reported the initial biochemical studies on venom from *C. sculpturatus*. The crude venom gives positive reactions to several tests for proteins, negative reactions to tests for polysaccharides and shows absorption spectra which are characteristic for proteins or peptides. The toxic principle was slowly inactivated in heat inactivation

*This work was supported in part by Grant NB-05535 from the National Institute of Neurological Diseases and Stroke, U.S. Public Health Service.

**Present address: USPHS Fellow. Laboratory of Neurological Research, University of Southern California School of Medicine, Los Angeles, California.

†Present address: Department of Biochemistry, School of Medicine, The Creighton Univeristy, Omaha, Nebraska.

studies. Separation of several components was achieved by chromatographing the crude venom on diethylaminoethyl (DEAE)-cellulose. Gel diffusion studies indicated that a multicomponent system was present in the toxic fraction.

McIntosh and Watt studied some of the biochemical and immunochemical aspects of *C. sculpturatus* venom. The crude venom was found to be stable over a wide range of pH and to resist digestion by proteolytic enzymes. Immunoelectrophoretic analysis indicated the presence of 10 precipitin bands.

This paper is a continuation of studies on the venom from *C. sculpturatus* and describes the purification of toxins from this scorpion.

MATERIALS

Venom was obtained by electrical stimulation of the telson of animals collected in Arizona. The venom was stored as a lyophilized powder at $-30°$ C. Carboxymethylcellulose (CMC) used was CM II, W. and R. Balston, Ltd., with a nominal capacity of 0.6 milli-equivalents per gram. Amberlite resin CG-50, 200–400 mesh, was obtained from Mallinckrodt. Fisher Scientific supplied Cleland's reagent. Mann Research Laboratories was the source of O-Iodosobenzoic acid. The immunoelectrophoresis apparatus was obtained from LKB (Sweden). All chemicals were of analytical grade. Solutions were made with distilled-deionized water.

METHODS

All chromatography was done at 4 to $8°$ C in a Gilson refrigerated fraction collector. Chromatographic procedures were conducted with standard commercial glass columns fitted with sintered glass supports. Ammonium acetate (NH_4 Ac) buffers were used. These solutions were adjusted to the desired pH by addition of either concentrated NH_4 OH or acetic acid.

The venom was dissolved in the starting buffer and centrifuged at 6,000 RPM for 10–15 minutes to remove insoluble material. Flow rates were controlled by a peristaltic pump (Holter Co., Bridgeport, Pa.). All samples were analyzed spectrophotometrically for their protein concentration at 280 mμ.

Determination of toxicity

LD_{50} of the venom was calculated according to the procedure of Reed and Muench (1938). Venom and toxic fractions were dissolved in water and injected subcutaneously into 18–20 g albino mice. Purified fractions generally were stabilized by addition of bovine serum albumin for a total protein concentration of 2.0 mg/ml. Toxicity tests on the isolated neuro-toxins were done with solutions of unknown concentrations. Purification of the neurotoxins was determined by locating the toxic peaks after each stage of separation.

Chromatography on CMC and amberlite CG-50

The CMC was precycled and regenerated according to the manufacturer's procedure. Amberlite CG-50 resin, 200–400 mesh, was cycled and treated generally following the method of Hirs (1955). The slurry was suspended in water and titrated to the desired pH with NH_4OH or acetic acid, then washed and suspended in starting buffer. A column 2.0 X 39.0 cm was poured and flow rates of 10.0 ml per hour maintained with a peristaltic pump. The amount of the CMC toxic fraction chromatographed was 75.0 mg. Elution was carried out using a linear gradient prepared by allowing 650.0 ml of 0.3 M NH_4Ac, pH 6.8 to flow into a reservoir containing 650.0 ml of 0.1 M NH_4Ac, pH 6.8. Continuous mixing was maintained with a magnetic mixer.

Fraction i, obtained from the linear gradient elution, was concentrated and subjected to equilibrium chromatography on Amberlite. A 13.0 mg sample of fraction i was chromatographed on a column 1.25 X 17.0 cm and eluted with 0.1 M NH_4Ac, pH 6.8. The remaining protein obtained from the linear gradient chromatography was concentrated and chromatographed on an Amberlite column 1.25 X 23.0 cm with 0.1 M NH_4Ac, pH 6.8. Three fractions were obtained from this procedure and identified as fractions 2, 3, and 4. Fraction 3 (17.0 mg) was then chromatographed on an Amberlite column 1.25 X 18.0 cm using a stepwise elution procedure. The buffer was changed to 0:2 M NH_4Ac, pH 6.8 after eluting with 100 ml of the starting buffer. Fractions 2 and 4 were not chromatographed further. All four fractions were lethal and identified in the order of their elution as toxins I, II, III and IV.

In a separate purification procedure, 30.0 mg of a CMC fraction was subjected to equilibrium chromatography on Amberlite CG-50 using 0.1 M NH_4Ac, pH 6.8 as the buffer. Five milliliter fractions were collected. Flow rate was maintained at 10–15 ml per hour. Other conditions were the same as previously described.

Isoelectric pH studies

Immunoelectrophoresis was used in order to conserve toxin. Determinations were done with a standard immunoelectrophoresis apparatus. Toxins I, III and IV were electrophoresed at pH 8.6, 10.0 and 10.6. Sodium barbital (veronal) and glycine-NaOH buffers, 0.08 M, were used. A 1.0 per cent solution of Noble agar was prepared with each buffer containing merthiolate (1:10,000) as a preservative. Toxins I, III and IV were electrophoresed for 45 minutes at 250 volts. The troughs were then charged with 100 μl of anti-venom sera and incubated at 25° C overnight.

Electrophoresis on cellulose acetate

Toxins I and III were electrophoresed on cellulose acetate at pH 8.6 and 11.0 using 0.08 M barbital and 0.09 M β-alanine buffer. Two different electro-phoretic conditions were used: with barbital buffer, the toxins were electro-phoresed for 45 minutes at 300 volts and with β-alanine, for one hour at 345 volts.

Cellulose polyacetate strips (Sepraphore III) was the carrier. The strips were heated for 10 minutes at 100° C after the electrophoretic run to fix the protein. The strips were then stained with amido black for 10 minutes and cleared with a 5 per cent acetic acid solution.

Immunoelectrophoresis of amberlite fractions

The same conditions as those described under isoelectric pH studies were used. Toxins I, III and IV were subjected to analysis by immunoelectro-phoresis. The troughs were charged with either crude venom antiserum or rabbit antisera prepared against toxins I and III.

Qualitative determination of sulfhydryl and disulfide groups

Three different concentrations of Cleland's reagent (dithiothreitol) were checked for their effects on the crude venom. The final reagent concentra-tions after addition to the venom were 10^{-1}, 10^{-3} and 2×10^{-2} M. The final venom concentration was 1.10 mg/ml. Venom and dithiothreitol were prepared in 0.1 M, pH 7.5 tris buffer. Toxicity was checked after 30 minutes treatment at 25° C.

O-Iodosobenzoic acid (Na) was prepared in 0.05 M citrate buffer, pH 3.8. Venom concentration was 2.0 mg/ml water. One-half milliliter of the reagent was added to 0.5 ml venom; the final reagent concentration was 10^{-2} M and the final venom concentration was 1.0 mg/ml. The mixture was reacted at 25° C and toxicity was checked after 1.5 and 24 hours.

Amino acid composition

Samples (1.0 mg) of each toxin were digested in 6.0 N HCl for 20 and 40 hours in sealed evacuated tubes (Moore and Stein, 1963). Two analyses were done using duplicate samples of each toxin. Hydrolysates were analyzed in an amino acid analyzer, Spinco model M5 (Beckman, Spinco Division). Column flow rate was 50 ml per hour. Corrections were made for losses of serine, threonine and tyrosine incurred during hydrolysis. Corrections for loss of halfcystine were based on recovery data for insulin. Tryptophan residue determinations were done separately according to the spectrophotometric method of Beaven and Holiday (1952). Samples were read in a Beckman model DB spectrophotometer and the absorption spectra plotted on an integrated power driven Speedomax G recorder.

RESULTS

Isolation of the toxins

In the initial purification scheme, 153.0 mg of venom was chromatographed on CMC (Figure 1). Lethality was located in tubes 232–260. Figure 2 shows results obtained by subjecting this fraction to equilibrium chromatography on Amberlite CG-50. Four peaks were obtained and all were lethal at the concentrations tested. The four toxic peaks were arbitrarily identified in the order of their elution as toxins I, II, III, and IV.

In a second experiment 429.0 mg sample of venom was then chromatographed on CMC (Figure 3). Lethality was located in tubes 610–700. This toxic fraction was then chromatographed on an Amberlite column. Figure 4 shows the elution pattern obtained by using a linear gradient from 0.1 M to 0.3 M NH_4 Ac at pH 6.8. Two fractions were collected representing tubes 145–163 and 164–232 respectively. Fraction 1, containing 13.60 O.D. units, was concentrated and subjected to equilibrium chromatography on Amberlite CG-50 with 0.1 M NH_4 Ac, pH 6.8. The resulting peak is shown in Figure 5 and was identified as toxin I.

The tubes remaining from the above gradient elution were concentrated

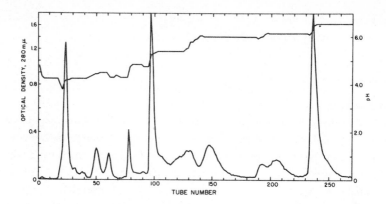

FIGURE 1. *Centruroides sculpturatus* venom (153.0 mg) chromatographed on carboxymethylcellulose (CMC). A discontinuous elution scheme with NH_4Ac buffer was used. Lethality is located in tubes 232–260

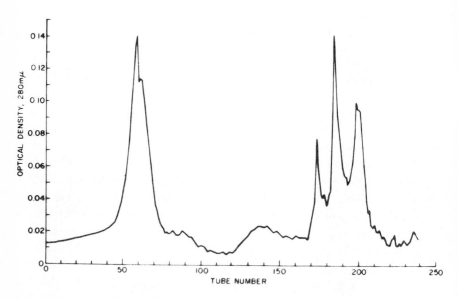

FIGURE 2. Elution profile of the toxic fraction in Figure 1 chromatographed on Amberlite CG-50 with 0.1 M NH_4Ac, pH 6.8. All four peaks are lethal

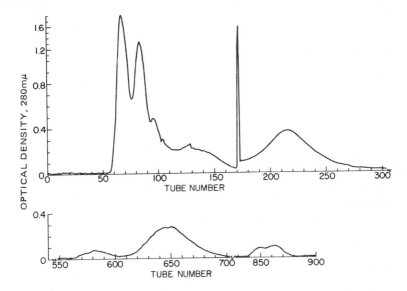

FIGURE 3.   *C. sculpturatus* venom (429.0 mg) separated on CMC using discontinuous chromatography with NH$_4$Ac. Lethality is located in tubes 610–700

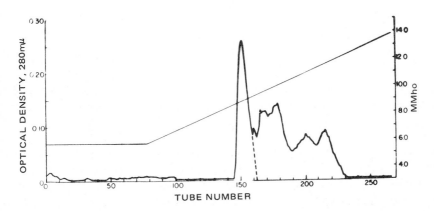

FIGURE 4.   Linear gradient elution of the toxic fraction in Figure 3 on Amberlite CG-50. The gradient was from 0.1 to 0.3 M NH$_4$Ac, pH 6.8

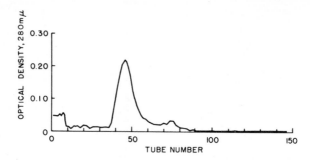

FIGURE 5.   Fraction 1 (tubes 145–163) in Figure 4 subjected to equilibrium chromatography on Amberlite with 0.1 M NH$_4$Ac, pH 6.8. The above peak was identified as Toxin I

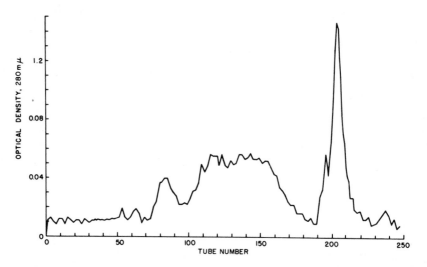

FIGURE 6.   Fraction 2 (tubes 164–232) in Figure 4 subjected to equilibrium chromatography on Amberlite with 0.1 M NH$_4$Ac, pH 6.8. All three peaks were lethal

and again subjected to equilibrium chromatography on Amberlite CG-50. The toxins were eluted with 0.1 M NH$_4$Ac, pH 6.8. Figure 6 shows the elution pattern. Three toxic peaks were obtained and identified as fractions 2, 3 and 4. Fractions 2 (tubes 70-99) and 4 (tubes 190–220) were not chromatographed further and identified as toxins II and IV. Tubes 100–183 were concentrated and again chromatographed on Amberlite using equilibrium

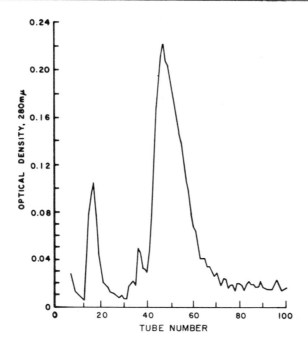

FIGURE 7.   Tubes 100–183 rechromatographed on Amberlite using equilibrium chromatography (0.1 M NH_4Ac, pH 6.8). The second peak was lethal and identified as toxin III

chromatography (Figure 7). A single toxic peak was obtained and identified as toxin III.

Toxcity tests of isolated toxins

The four toxins were tested for toxicity in mice. Concentrations of the toxins were about 1.0 mg/ml water. The toxins were administered subcutaneously and all four toxins produced death from a minimum of 8 minutes duration for toxin IV to 51 minutes for toxin II.

Qualitative determination of sulfhydryl and disulfide groups in venom

Dithiothreitol inactivated the venom. Five mice were tested at a level of 2.5 mg/kg with the dithiothreitol treated venom. None of the mice showed any ill effects. O-Iodosobenzoic acid had no effect on venom toxicity. A group of five mice treated at a concentration of 2.2 mg/kg died. Reagent controls in both cases were not toxic. Venom controls for the two reagents gave the following results: dithiothreitol, 5/5 deaths at 1.7 mg/kg; and O-Iodosobenzoic acid, 5/5 deaths at 2.2 mg/kg.

Isoelectric pH determination of purified toxins

The four purified toxins were examined immunoelectrophoretically to study their mobility characteristics at different pH values. Initially all four toxins were electrophoresed at pH 8.6 and found to migrate strongly as cations. Toxins I, III and IV were then electrophoresed at pH 10.0; all three toxins still migrated as cations. Finally toxins I and IV were found to migrate as cations at pH 10.6. Toxins II and III were not checked at this pH. The toxins were not examined above 10.6.

Electrophoresis on cellulose acetate

Toxins I and III were analyzed by electrophoresis on cellulose acetate at pH 8.6 and 11.0. Both toxins migrated as cations. A single band was observed for each toxin indicating the presence of a single component.

Analysis of purified toxins by immunoelectrophoresis

Toxins I and IV were electrophoresed in buffered agar and reacted against rabbit antivenom. Only one precipitin band was present for each toxin. Crude scorpion venom was then electrophoresed under the same conditions and reacted with either anti-toxin I or -toxin III rabbit serum. Again only one precipitin band was visible for each toxin. Specific antisera were not available for toxins II and IV.

Amino acid composition studies

Table 1 shows the amino acid composition of the four toxins. The results represent two different analyses. Results were obtained by averaging the values of duplicate samples from 20 and 40 hour hydrolysis. The values indicated for serine and threonine are extrapolated values. Methionine is absent in all four toxins. Alanine is missing from toxins I and II; isoleucine is missing from toxins III and IV. The total number of amino acid residues

TABLE 1   Amino acid composition of the toxins from *C. sculpturatus*

| Amino Acid | Molar Ratio[a] | | | |
	Toxin I	Toxin II	Toxin III	Toxin IV
Lysine	8.79 (9)	9.55 (10)	8.03 (8)	8.92 (9)
Histidine	1.00 (1)	1.00 (1)	1.00 (1)	1.00 (1)
Amide NH$_3$[b]				
Arginine	1.06 (1)	0.90 (1)	1.86 (2)	2.38 (2)
Aspartic Acid	6.93 (7)	5.47 (5)	7.09 (7)	7.42 (7)
Threonine[c]	5.00 (5)	5.00 (5)	4.00 (4)	1.00 (1)
Serine[c]	2.00 (2)	6.00 (6)	2.00 (2)	4.00 (4)
Glutamic Acid	6.03 (6)	4.72 (5)	7.51 (8)	9.04 (9)
Proline	3.59 (4)	2.59 (3)	2.94 (3)	2.11 (2)
Glycine	10.44 (10)	8.58 (9)	8.86 (9)	9.38 (9)
Alanine	0	0	2.77 (3)	4.35 (4)
Half-Cystine[d]	7.75 (8)	4.84 (6)	6.70 (8)	6.38 (8)
Valine	1.15 (1)	0.66 (1)	3.08 (3)	3.08 (3)
Methionine	0	0	0	0
Isoleucine	1.04 (1)	0.82 (1)	0	0
Leucine	4.71 (5)	3.31 (3)	6.21 (6)	7.72 (8)
Tyrosine	6.33 (6)	4.10 (4)	7.99 (8)	6.80 (7)
Phenylalanine	2.20 (2)	1.92 (4)	2.59 (3)	1.40 (1)
Tryptophan[e]	2.19 (2)	1.99 (2)	3.12 (3)	3.43 (3)
Total	70	64	78	78

a/ Taking histidine = 1.0. Numbers in parentheses represent the closest integer.
b/ Not determined. c/ Extropolated values. d/ Based on recovery in insulin.
e/ Determined spectrophotometrically.

present in the purified toxins are presented in Table 1. The total residue varies from 64 for toxin II to 78 residues for toxins III and IV.

Table 2 presents the minimum molecular weights of the purified toxins. The minimum molecular weights were calculated from the number of amino acid residues present for each toxin. The values given represent the sum total of the residue weight for each amino acid.

Table 3 presents the amino acid composition of the neurotoxins from *C. sculpturatus* and *Androctonus australis* for comparative purposes.

Criteria of homogeneity

Homogeneity of the purified toxins was demonstrated by the following. (1) Toxin I and III eluted from equilibrium chromatography on Amberlite CG-50

TABLE 2 The minimum molecular weights of the toxins from *C. sculpturatus*

Amino Acid	Residue Weight	Toxin I	Toxin II	Toxin III	Toxin IV
Lysine	128.19	1153.71 (9)	1281.90 (10)	1025.52 (8)	1153.71(9)
Histidine	137.16	137.16 (1)	127.16 (1)	137.16 (1)	137.16 (1)
Amide NH$_3$	16.02	0	0	0	0
Arginine	156.21	156.21 (1)	156.21 (1)	312.42 (2)	312.42 (2)
Aspartic Acid	115.11	805.77 (7)	575.55 (5)	805.77 (7)	805.77 (7)
Threonine	101.11	505.55 (5)	505.55 (5)	404.44 (4)	101.11 (1)
Serine	87.10	174.20 (2)	522.60 (6)	174.20 (2)	348.40 (4)
Glutamic Acid	129.13	774.78 (6)	645.65 (5)	1033.04 (8)	1162.17 (9)
Proline	97.13	388.52 (4)	291.39 (3)	291.39 (3)	194.26 (2)
Glycine	57.07	570.70 (10)	513.63 (9)	513.63 (9)	513.63 (9)
Alanine	71.10	0	0	213.30 (3)	284.40 (4)
Half-Cystine	101.15	809.20 (8)	606.90 (6)	809.20 (8)	809.20 (8)
Valine	99.15	99.15 (1)	99.15 (1)	297.45 (3)	297.45 (3)
Methionine	131.21	0	0	0	0
Isolecuine	113.17	113.17 (1)	113.17 (1)	0	0
Leucine	113.17	565.85 (5)	339.51 (3)	679.02 (6)	905.36 (8)
Tyrosine	163.19	979.14 (6)	652.76 (4)	1305.52 (8)	1142.33 (7)
Phenylalanine	147.19	294.38 (2)	294.38 (2)	441.57 (3)	147.19 (1)
Tryptophan	186.22	372.44 (2)	372.44 (2)	558.66 (3)	558.66 (3)
Minimum Molecular Weight		7900	7108	9002	8873

Numbers in parentheses represent the closest integer.

as symmetrical peaks. (2) Toxin I and III migrated as single bands on cellulose acetate at pH 8.6 and 11.0. (3) All four toxins gave single precipitin bands in agar when reacted against antivenom sera. (4) Toxin I and III antiserum gave single precipitin bands when reacted against unfractionated venom. (5) Amino acid composition data shows that methionine is absent from all four toxins. (6) In addition, alanine is missing from toxin I and II and isoleucine from toxin III and IV.

DISCUSSION

Purification procedures of the toxins of *C. sculpturatus* described in this paper differ from earlier studies (Watt, 1964; McIntosh and Watt, 1967),

TABLE 3   The amno acid composition of the toxins from *C. sculpturatus* and *Androctorus australis* for comparative purposes

| Amino Acid | *C. sculpturatus*[a] | | | | *A. australis*[b] | |
	Toxin I	*Toxin II*	*Toxin III*	*Toxin IV*	*Toxin I*	*Toxin II*
Lysine	9	10	8	9	6	5
Histidine	1	1	1	1	1	2
Amide NH_3[c]	—	—	—	—	2	6
Arginine	1	1	2	2	2	3
Aspartic Acid	7	5	7	7	9	8
Threonine	5	5	4	1	2	3
Serine	2	6	2	4	6	2
Glutamic Acid	6	5	8	9	0	4
Proline	4	3	3	2	6	3
Glycine	10	9	9	9	6	7
Alanine	0	0	3	4	1	3
Half-Cystine	8	6	8	8	8	8
Valine	1	1	3	3	4	4
Methionine	0	0	0	0	0	0
Isoleucine	1	1	0	0	3	1
Leucine	5	3	6	8	4	2
Tyrosine	6	4	8	7	3	7
Phenylalanine	2	2	3	1	1	1
Tryptophan	2	2	3	3	1	1
Total	70	64	78	78	64	64
Minimum Molecular Weight	7900	7108	9002	8873	6822	7249

[a] Taking histidine = 1.0.
[b] Taking phenylalanine = 1.0.
[c] Not determined.

utilizing chromatography on DEAE-cellulose. Purification of the toxins was achieved essentially using two steps: (1) discontinuous chromatography on CMC and (2) chromatography on Amberlite CG-50 using gradient elution, discontinuous elution and equilibrium chromatography.

The CMC fraction was considerably less toxic at low concentrations than when stabilized with bovine serum albumin. These results are in agreement with data reported for *A. australis* (Rochat *et al.*, 1967). Whether or not the loss of activity is due to molecular disassociation as has been suggested for the neurotoxins of *A. australis* (Rochat *et al.*, 1967) is not known. Toxicity of the purified toxins was checked in mice. All four toxins were found to be lethal. The purified toxins were not subjected to stability tests. Tests to identify the toxins from *C. sculpturatus* as specific neurotoxins have not been done. It is expected that these proteins will exhibit neurotoxic activity similar to that described for the neurotoxins of *A. australis*.

General studies of the electrophoretic behaviour of the isolated toxins indicate they may have a rather high pH_i. Preliminary indications are that the pH_i values are probably 9 or above. Confirmation of the electrophoretic data for *C. sculpturatus* is yet to be done. However, the high electrophoretic values correlate with the high pH_i found for the toxins of *A. australis* and *B. occitanus* (Miranda *et al.*, 1964a; 1964b). In view of the relatively large number of lysine residues present in the toxins, a high pH_i might be expected.

The isolated toxins were shown to be homogeneous by equilibrium chromatography (symmetrical curve), electrophoresis on cellulose acetate and analysis by immunoelectrophoresis using venom antisera, and anti-toxin I and III serum. Homogeneity was also supported by amino acid composition studies. All four toxins were found to be lacking two amino acids each.

Amino acid composition studies indicate that a certain amount of similarity exists between the toxins of *C. sculpturatus* and the amino acid composition data published for *A. australis* (Rochat *et al.*, 1967). Methionine is absent from the toxins of *C. sculpturatus* and *A. australis*. The possible absence of methionine from the toxins was previously indicated by the negative results obtained with O-Iodosobenzoic acid, a sulfhydryl group specific reagent. The possibility that sulfur was present in the toxins as cystine was indicated by results obtained with dithiothreitol, a disulfide group specific reagent. No activity was demonstrable in venom treated with this reagent. Six to 8 residues of half-cystine are present which correlates with the high sulfur content of *A. australis* toxins.

Alanine is missing in toxins I and II while toxins III and IV have 3 and 4 residues respectively. Isoleucine is not present in toxins III and IV but toxins I and II each have one residue. Alanine and isoleucine are present in both toxins of *A. australis*. Glutamic acid is absent in toxin I of *A. australis* but is present in all four toxins from *C. sculpturatus*. High amounts of aromatic amino acids are present: 10 residues for toxins I and II; 14 residues in toxin III; and 11 residues in toxin IV.

Size of the toxins range from 64 to 78 amino acid residues. Toxin II is the smallest with 64 amino acid residues. Toxin III and IV each have 78 residues.

The minimum molecular weights are: toxin I–7900; toxin II–7108; toxin III–9002; toxin IV–8873.

Aberrant forms of toxins were observed in *A. australis* and *B. occitanus* (Miranda *et al.*, 1966b; Rochat *et al.*, 1967). These aberrant forms were reported to be a result of non-specific association of the toxins with contaminating proteins. According to Rochat *et al.* (1967) chromatography on DEAE-Sephadex after chromatography on Amberlite is necessary to dissociate ionic complexes of the toxins with glycopeptides. It has not been determined if the four toxins in *C. sculpturatus* represent four true toxins, molecular variants or one or more aberrant forms.

It should be emphasized that the amino acid composition data represent preliminary results. These data should not be interpreted as representing exhaustive analyses. Insufficient amounts of purified toxins preclude additional analyses at this time. Therefore, some changes in composition of the four toxins may be eventually observed.

SUMMARY

The venom of *Centruroides sculpturatus* contains four toxins (I, II, III, and IV). Purification was achieved by initial separation on carboxymethyl-cellulose followed by gradient elution, discontinuous and equilibrium chromatography on Amberlite CG-50. Homogeneity was demonstrated by equilibrium chromatography on Amberlite, electrophoresis on cellulose acetate, immunoelectrophoresis using anti-venom sera and anti-toxin I and -toxin III serum, and supported by amino acid composition studies. Preliminary examination indicates a pH_i value above 8.6 for the toxins.

Amino acid composition studies show that methionine is absent from all four toxins. Alanine is missing from toxins I and II; isoleucine is absent in toxins III and IV. Toxin I has 70 amino acids; toxin II, 64; and toxins III and IV each have 78 amino acids. Minimum molecular weights based on amino acid composition studies are: toxin I–7900; toxin II–7108; toxin III–9002; and toxin IV–8873. It is unknown at present if these toxins represent true molecular types, molecular variants or one or more aberrant forms.

References

Beaven, G. H. and E. R. Holiday 1952 'Ultraviolet absorption spectra of proteins and amino acids,' In: Anson, M. L. (ed.), *Advances in Protein Chemistry*, 7: 319. Academic Press, New York.

Hirs, C. H. W. 1955 'Chromatography of enzymes on ion exchange resins.' In: Colowick, S. P. and N. O. Kaplan (eds.), *Methods in Enzymology*. Vol. 1, p. 113. Academic Press, New York.

McIntosh, M. E. and D. D. Watt 1967 'Biochemical-immunochemical aspects of the venom from the scorpion *Centruroides sculpturatus.*' In: Russell, F. E. and P. R. Saunders (eds.), *Animal Toxins.* p. 47. Pergamon Press, Oxford.

Miranda, F. and S. Lissitzky 1961 'Scorpamines: the toxic proteins of scorpion venoms.' *Nature*, 190: 443.

Miranda, F., H. Rochat and S. Lissitzky 1964a 'Sur les neurotoxines de deux especes de scorpions Nord-Africaines.' *Toxicon*, 2: 51.

Miranda, R., H. Rochat and S. Lissitzky, 1964b 'Sur les neurotoxines de deux especes de scorpions Nord-Africains. II. Properties des neurotoxines (Scorpamines) d'*Androctonus australis* (L.) et de *Buthus occitanus* (Am.)'. *Toxicon*, 2: 113.

Miranda, F., H. Rochat, C. Rochat and S. Lissitzky 1966a 'Essais de purification des neurotoxines du venin d'un scorpion d' Amerique du Sud (*Tityus serrulatus* L. et M.) par des methodes chromatographiques.' *Toxicon*, 4: 145.

Miranda, F., H. Rochat, Ch. Rochat and S. Lissitzky 1966b 'Complexes moleculaiaes presentes par les neurotoxines animales. I. Neurotoxines des venins de scorpions (*Androctonus australis Hector* et *Buthus occitanus tunetanus*).' *Toxicon*, 4: 123.

Moore, S. and W. Stein 1963 'Chromatographic determination of amino acid by the use of automatic recording equipment.' In: Colowick, S. P. and N. O. Kaplan (eds.), *Methods in Enzymology*, Vol. VI, p. 819. Academic Press, New York.

Reed, L. J. and H. Muench 1938 'A Simple method of estimating fifty per cent endpoints.' *Am. J. Hyg.*, 27: 493.

Rochat, C., H. Rochat, F. Miranda and S. Lissitzky 1967 'Purification and some properties of the neurotoxines of *Androctonus australis Hector.*' *Biochemistry*, 6: 578.

Watt, D. D. 1964 'Biochemical studies of the venom from the scorpion *Centruroides sculpturatus.*' *Toxicon*, 2: 171.

RECENT DEVELOPMENTS IN THE CHEMISTRY OF MARINE TOXINS

P. J. SCHEUER

Department of Chemistry, University of Hawaii,
Honolulu, Hawaii

RESEARCH ON THE CHEMISTRY of marine toxins came into its own in 1964 when the structure of tetrodotoxin, the toxic principle isolated from the ovaries of puffer fish, was determined independently in four laboratories (Mosher *et al.,* 1964; Woodward 1964; Goto *et al.,* 1965; Tsuda, 1966). Since that time we have seen the elucidation of the structure of pahutoxin, the toxic secretion of the boxfish (Boylan and Scheuer, 1967), and the structural determination of several of the holothurins, the triterpenoid glycosides isolated from sea cucumbers (Chanley *et al.,* 1966). In this paper I will summarize some recently published research on the holothurins and will mention several of the problems which are currently under investigation in my laboratory. This will cover some aspects of the chemistry of the toxins isolated from sea hare digestive glands, of ciguatoxin, and of palytoxin.

THE HOLOTHURINS

The occurrence of toxic saponins in sea cucumbers (holothurins) has been known for some time (Nigrelli and Jakowska, 1960). The sea cucumbers constitute one of the five classes of animals in the phylum Echinodermata. The other classes are the sea urchins (echinoids), the brittle stars (ophiuroids), the sea stars (asteroids), and the sea lilies (crinoids).

I

Initial work by Chanley *et al.* (1959) has established that some of the glycosides isolated from the Cuverian glands of the Bahamian sea cucumber *Actinopyga agassizi* may be precipitated as a cholesterol complex. This particular mixture was designated holothurin A. Holothurin A was further recognized as a mixture of aglycones, which are linked to four sugar molecules and a molecule of sulphuric acid as the sodium salt. The sugars were identified as D-xylose, D-glucose, 3-0-methyl-D-glucose and D-quinovose. The sugar sequence was established by Chanley *et al.* (1960) through enzymatic hydrolysis of holothurin A with an extract of *Helix pomatia* at pH 5.2. By periodic paper chromatographic analysis of the hydrolysate over 189 hr it was found that the sequence is in the order aglycone-D-xylose-D-glucose-3-0-methyl-D-glucose-D-quinovose. The sulfate residue was found to be linked to xylose.

The structures of two of the aglycones, which comprised 30 percent of the total mixture, have been determined by Chanley *et al.* (1966). The name holothurinogenin has been adopted for the parent compound and, based on this nomenclature, the two aglycones are 22,25-oxidoholothurinogenin (I) 17-deoxy-22,25-oxidoholothurinogenin.

The structures of several closely related compounds have been elucidated in other laboratories (Tursch *et al.*, 1967; Roller *et al.*, 1969; Habermehl and Volkwein, 1970; Tursch *et al.*, 1970) and the parent structure has been rigorously correlated with that of lanosterol (Roller *et al.*, 1969).

It had been recognized that at least the diene system and perhaps other features of the holothurinogenin structure arose during acid hydrolysis of the glycosides since the intact mixture lacks the characteristic UV absorption of the diene system. Chanley and Rossi (1969) by enzymatic hydrolysis of

II

desulfated holothurin A, established the structure of the native aglycone and designated it 22,25-oxido*neo* holothurinogenin (II).

Shimada (1969) recently isolated from the body wall of the sea cucumber *Stichopus japonicus*, an antifungal constituent which he named holotoxin. He assumes this compound to be a steroidal glycoside different from the known holothurins.

Hashimoto and coworkers (Hashimoto and Yasumoto, 1960; Yasumoto and Hashimoto, 1965, 1967; Yasumoto *et al.*, 1966) investigated other classes in the phylum Echinodermata for the occurrence of toxic glycosides. They discovered similar compounds only in the sea stars and named these compounds asterosaponins. These substances seemed to differ from the holothurins both in the aglycone structure and in the sugar components. So far only the sugar components have been determined.

SEA HARE TOXINS

Sea hares, members of the family Aplysiidae, class Gastropoda, have had a reputation of being toxic since antiquity (Halstead, 1965). Among the esoteric properties ascribed to sea hares was its ability to abort the fetus of a pregnant woman who would look at sea hare. The first attempt at a modern scientific investigation was made by Flury in 1915. He describes three secretions derived from the Mediterranean sea hare, *Aplysia depilans*: an unpleasantly smelling colorless fluid secreted by the skin; a white viscous liquid secreted by an 'opaline' gland; and a purple secretion also originating

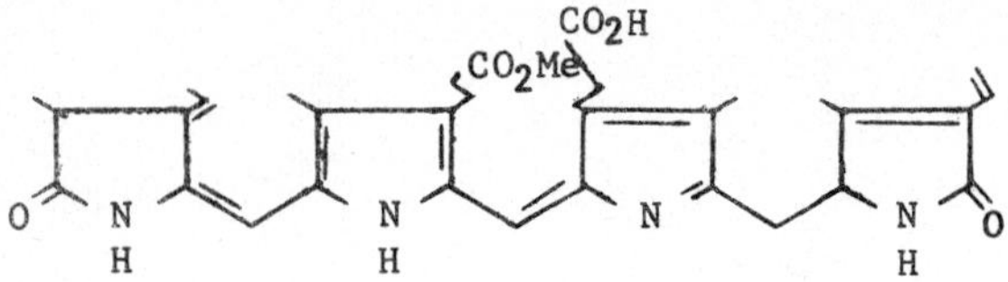

III

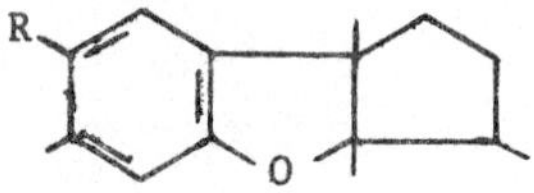

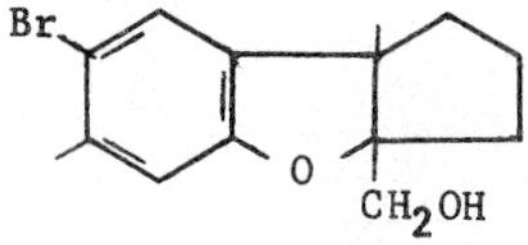

IV   R = Br

V   R = H

VI

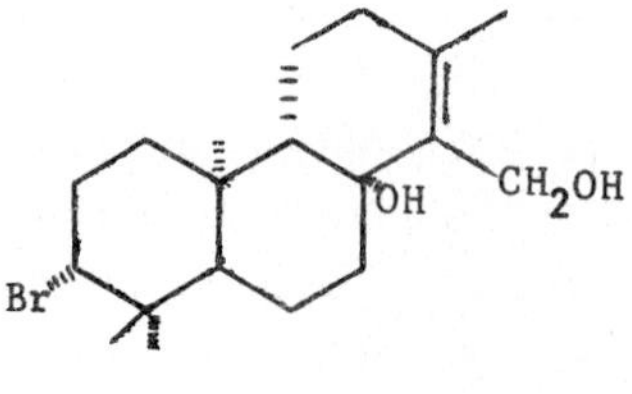

VII

from a gland. The opaline fluid had a bitter taste, produced an eye irritation in rabbits and dogs, and caused muscular paralysis when injected into coelenterates, annelids, frogs, and other cold-blooded animals.

Winkler *et al.* in 1962 prepared an acetone extract of the digestive glands of the sea hares *A. californica* and *A. vaccaria*. They called this extract aplysin and studied its pharmacology. These workers found neuromuscular activity reminiscent of choline esters. They noted respiratory distress, excitement and death some five min after i.p. injection. However, further *in vivo* and *in vitro* studies were somewhat contradictory.

The purple pigment of *A. limacina* was recently studied by Rüdiger (1967) and its structure (III) was elucidated.

TABLE 1.   Relative Toxicity of Some Sea Hare Digestive Glands

Species	Toxicity Rating
Hawaii	
Aplysia dactylomela	—
A. juliana	—
A. pulmonica	+
Dolabella auricularia	++
D. scapula	+
Dolabrifera dolabrifera	++
Stylocheilus longicauda	++
Japan	
Aplysia kurodai	+
Dolabella auricularia	+

Hirata and coworkers in Japan (Yamamura and Hirata, 1963) studied the ether extracts of whole dried specimens of *Aplysia kurodai*. After saponification, extraction, and chromatography they isolated and characterized aplysin, and aplysinol, have also been found by Irie *et al.* (1969) in algae of debromoaplysin (V), and aplysinol (VI).

Racemic aplysin and racemic debromoaplysin have been synthesized (25). A fourth bromo compound, aplysin-20 (VII) a diterpene, was also isolated from the same animals (Matsuda *et al.*, 1967).

It is interesting to note that the three sesquiterpenes, aplysin, debromoaplysin, and aplysinol, have also been found by Irie *et al.* (1969) in algae of the genus *Laurencia*.

In our own work we surveyed a number of sea hares in order to check whether toxicity of digestive glands was a common property. The results are summarized in Table 1.

It may be seen that two species of *Aplysia* showed no toxicity at all, while the toxicity of four other species was only modest. Furthermore, one species, *D. auricularia* showed greater toxicity in specimens collected in Hawaii than in Japan.

We have been able to isolate identical toxins from *A. pulmonica* and from *Stylocheilus longicauda*. Initially, the acetone extract of the digestive glands was partitioned between ether and water. Each phase contains a toxin. Both toxins have been evaluated pharmacologically (Watson, 1969), but all chemical work has so far been carried out with the ether-soluble toxin.

The symptoms of mice which follow i.p. injection of the water-soluble toxin include convulsions, respiratory distress, salivation, and sudden death. The salient pharmacological responses of this toxin include mild bradycardia, hypotension, and decreased respiratory rate. Symptoms caused by the ether-soluble toxin include hypersensitivity, viciousness, paralysis, and slow death, while the pharmacological responses include bradycardia, hypertension and increased respiratory rate.

The ether-soluble toxin was initially purified by silicic acid chromatography and the toxic fraction was eluted from the column with 1–5% of methanol in chloroform. Further purification was achieved by dry column chromatography, gel filtration, and eventually thin-layer chromatography. This yielded a homogeneous toxic fraction, MLD 0.3 mg/kg in a yield of 90 ppm. Mild acetylation followed by thin-layer chromatography led to the separation of the product into three acetates with the molecular formulas $C_{36}H_{49}O_{11}Br$ and two isomeric acetates of composition $C_{36}H_{50}O_{11}$. All three acetates appeared to be diacetates, which renders the molecular formulas of the parent compounds $C_{32}H_{45}O_9Br$ and $C_{32}H_{46}O_9$.

From *A. pulmonica* alone we have isolated a non-toxic companion substance which travels closely with the toxin; this substance is nitrogeneous and has the composition $C_{28}H_{45}N_3O_5$.

CIGUATOXIN

Among the human intoxications which are caused by marine organisms and described in the literature, the disease known as ciguatera stands out as a puzzling phenomenon. Many factors contribute to the puzzle. Although the disease is rarely fatal, it contributes heavily to the public health and nutritional problems of all people who depend on reef fish for part or most of their protein food. This includes the inhabitants of many of the archipelagoes in the tropical Pacific and Caribbean as well as the Great Barrier Reef of northern Australia. The neurological and gastrointestinal symptoms in man are often bizarre and include loss of motor ability and reversal of temperature sensations besides vomiting and diarrhoea. Many species of fish have been implicated at one time or another, but snappers (Lutjanidae) groupers (Serranidae), moray eels (Muraenidae), and surgeon fishes (Acanthuridae) are perhaps the most frequent bearers of this toxin. In addition to the variability of symptoms and the variability of involved fish species, the geographical incidents of ciguatera is also variable. An island group with no prior history of ciguatera may suddenly become toxic and gradually decline in toxicity, or only one reef of an island may harbor toxic fish. The most comprehensive description of ciguatera has been rendered by Halstead (1967) in Vol. II of his work. More recently, the ecological and geographical parameters of ciguatera have been critically examined by Helfrich *et al.* (1968) and by Helfrich and Banner (1968). The most complete clinical and epidemiological study to-date has been reported from French Polynesia by Bagnis (1967).

Most of our recent work has been concentrated on the toxin isolated from the flesh of the moray eel, *Gymnothorax javanicus*. The eel flesh is cooked briefly and extracted with acetone. The acetone extract is concentrated and the aqueous residue is partitioned between water and ether. The toxin is found in the ether phase and is further purified by silicic acid chromatography, column and thin layer, followed by gel filtration on Sephadex. This yields a homogeneous toxin MLD, 0.025 mg/kg, in yields of 1–10 ppm.

We have recently succeeded in preparing a crystalline mercury derivative of the intact toxin. We have further been able to form a crystalline mercury derivative of the aqueous fraction derived from mild acid or base hydrolysis of the toxin. When the mercury is removed from the adduct of the degradation product a colorless crystalline substance is obtained.

Mass spectral data indicate that the toxin, which has a molecular weight of ~1500, consists of a sizable hydrocarbon moiety and nitrogeneous fragments. The molecule contains 3–4 nitrogen atoms.

PALYTOXIN   (Moore and Scheuer, 1971)

Limu make o Hana (deadly seaweed of Hana) is the Hawaiian phrase for a toxic organism which Malo (1951) described as follows. '... in Muolea, in the district of Hana, grew a poisonous moss in a certain pool or pond close to the ocean. It was used to smear on the spear points to make them fatal... The moss is said to be of a reddish color and is still to be found. It grows nowhere else than at that one spot.' According to Hawaiian legend* there lived in the Hana district a man who always seemed to be busy planting and harvesting. Whenever the people in the neighborhood went fishing, upon their return one of the group was missing. This went on for some time without anyone having

*Manuscript notes by Katherine Livermore on file at B. P. Bishop Museum, Honolulu.

an explanation for the mysterious disappearances. At last the fishermen became suspicious of the man who tended his taro patch. They grabbed him, tore off his clothes, and discovered on his back the mouth of a shark. They killed and burned him and threw the ashes into the sea. At the spot where this happened, so goes the legend, the *limu* became toxic. The tidepool containing the toxic *limu* subsequently became *kapu* (taboo) to the Hawaiians. They would cover the *limu* with stones (Malo, 1951) and were very secretive about its location. They firmly belived that disaster would strike if anyone were to attempt to gather the toxic *limu*.

Our long interest in marine toxins and specifically in the biological origin of ciguateric fishes prompted us to try and locate the toxic *limu*. Through the efforts of Professor A. H. Banner and Dr P. Helfrich of the Hawaii Institute of Marine Biology and by an elaborate chain of informers the tidepool was located and a small collection of the toxic *limu* was made on 31 December, 1961. Local residents reminded the members of the field party of the ancient *kapu* and warned of impending misfortune. Coincidentally, on that same afternoon a fire of unknown origin destroyed the main building of the Hawaii Marine Laboratory at Coconut Island, Oahu.

The collection was preserved in ethanol and returned to the laboratory. One of the collectors who had numerous scratches and abrasions on his hands and feet noted malaise as a consequence of contact with the mucous secretions. The symptoms persisted and he saw a physician, who however was unfamiliar with the syndrome and administered symptomatic therapy. To check gross toxicity an aliquot of the supernatant solvent was evaporated and the residue was tested by i.p. injection in mice. Without a doubt the alcohol had become highly toxic since almost instantenous death occurred even after dilution of the sample over several orders of magnitude. Severe reaction to the toxin was later observed on a collecting trip to Tahiti when the mucous secretions came in contact with open cuts on the feet and ankles. Severe local pain around the wounds, dizziness, chills, and nausea lasted for a day.

Another case came to our attention through a physician practicing in Hilo, Hawaii who treated a patient for a persistent eye irritation and impaired vision caused by the mucous secretion of an organism later identified as *Palythoa tuberculosa*. The patient had been collecting opihi (a limpet) on the Kalapana coast at Kaumomoa, Hawaii, when the tool he was using to pry the shellfish off the rocks slipped into a growth of soft coral, causing some mucus to squirt into his eye.

Taxonomic examination of the toxic organism showed it not to be a *limu*. In fact it was not a plant but an animal of the phylum Coelenterata, order Zoantharia, family Zoanthidae**. Halstead (1965) does not list the family Zoanthidae among toxic coelenterates; this may well indicate that our discovery was the first demonstration of toxicity among the Zoanthidae. In a subsequent extensive search for other occurrences of toxic zoanthids we located small populations near the Blowhole on Oahu and at Kaumomoa, Hawaii (through the courtesy of Mr A. Cooper) as well as a large bed in the Papara district of Tahiti, French Polynesia (discovered by Dr P. Helfrich). Since then Attaway (1968) has reported on toxic *Palythoa caribaeorum* and *P. mammilosa* from Jamaica and the Bahamas, and Hashimoto *et al.* (1969) found toxic *P. tuberculosa* at Ishigaki island in the Ryukyus.

Palytoxin is isolated by initial extraction with aqueous ethanol. Pigments and other non-toxic materials are then removed with benzene and 1-butanol. The remaining aqueous ethanolic extract is desalted on polyethylene and finally purified by Sephadex chromatography. Much of this chromatography is carried out in buffered solutions so that a final desalting step on polyethylene leads to a homogeneous material, which appears as a white hygroscopic powder on freeze-drying. It is homogeneous in 9 paper and 6 thin layer systems as well as by countercurrent distributions. The LD_{50} of the pure toxin is 0.15 μg/kg by i.v. injection in mice. Yields have ranged from 5–270 ppm.

In its pharmacological activity palytoxin seems to parallel the cardiac glycosides although it appears to be at least 100 times more active than the most active of the cardiac glycosides both in terms of lethal dose and of minimum effective dose (Rayner, unpublished data).

Palytoxin has a characteristic UV spectrum with maxima at 233 and 263 nm. The most prominent infrared bands occur at 330, 2900, 1650 and 1060 cm^{-1}. The NMR spectrum is exceedingly complex and only a few singlets at high field are readily discernible. Palytoxin is optically active with a specific rotation $[\alpha]_D$ + 27°. The toxin is sensitive to acid and base. The molecular weight of palytoxin is at least 2,500 with a possible composition of

---

**Originally, the species was thought to be *Palythoa vestitus* Verrill, but a careful reinvestigation of the Hawaiian zoanthids by G. E. Walsh and R. E. Bowers (in preparation) makes the binomial uncertain at present.

$C_{120}H_{200}N_4O_{52}$. It contains no small repetitive units such as sugars or amino acids and we have been unable to prepare crystalline derivatives of the intact toxin.

Among many degradative schemes the most fruitful ones have been oxidative in nature. Although oxidation leads to a relatively large number of products, we have been able to crystallize several of these and we have characterized several others.

SUMMARY

Recent developments in the chemistry of the holothurins, of ciguatoxin, sea hare toxins, and palytoxin are discussed.

ACKNOWLEDGMENTS

It is a pleasure to acknowledge my coworkers who have carried out the unpublished work described here: Yoshinori Kato (sea hares), Wataru Takahashi (ciguatoxin), Richard E. Moore and M. Younus Sheikh (palytoxin).

References

Attaway, D. 1968 'Isolation and partial characterization of Caribbean palytoxin.' Ph. D. Dissertation, University of Oklahoma.

Bagnis, R. 1967 'Les empoisonnements par le poisson en Polynésie française: Etude clinique et épidémiologique.' *Rev. Hyg. Med. Soc.*, 15: 619.

Boylan, D. B. and P. J. Scheuer 1967 'Pahutoxin: A fish poison.' *Science*, 155: 52.

Chanley, J. D., R. Ledeen, J. Wax, R. F. Nigrelli and H. Sobotka 1959 'The isolation, properties, and sugar components of holothurin A.' *J. Amer Chem. Soc.*, 81: 5180

Chanley, J. D., T. Mezzetti and H. E. Sobotka 1966 'The holothurinogenins.' *Tetrahedron*, 22: 1857

Chanley, J. D., J. Perlstein, R. F. Nigrelli and H. Sobotka 1960 'Further studies on the structure of holothurin.' *Ann. N. Y. Acad. Sci.*, 90: 902.

Chanley, J. D. and C. Rossi 1969 'The neo-holothurinogenins. III. Neoholothurinogenins by enzymatic hydrolysis of desulfated holothurin A.' *Tetrahedron*, 25: 1911.

Flury, F. 1915 'Über das Aplysiengift.' *Arch. exp. Pathol. Pharmakol.*, 79: 250.

Goto, T., Y. Kishi, S. Takahashi and Y. Hirota 1965 'Tetrodotoxin.' *Tetrahedron*, 21: 2059.

Habermehl, G. and G. Volkwein 1970 'Über Gifte der mittelmeerischen Holothurien. II. Die Aglyca der Toxine von *Holothuria polii*.' *Justus Liebigs Ann. Chem.*, 731: 53.

Halstead, B. W. 1965 *'Poisonous and Venomous Marine Animals of the World.'* Vol. I. U.S. Government Printing Office, Washington, D.C.

Halstead, B. W. 1967 *'Poisonous and Venomous Marine Animals of the World.'* Vol. II. U.S. Government Printing Office, Washington, D.C.

Hashimoto, Y., N. Fusetani and S. Kimura 1969 'Aluterin: A toxin of filefish, *Alutera scripta*, probably originating from a zoantharian, *Palythoa tuberculosa*. *Bull. Jap. Soc. Sci. Fisheries*, 35: 1086.

Hashimoto, Y. and T. Yasumoto 1960 'Confirmation of saponin as a toxic principle of Star Fish,' *Bull. Jap. Soc. Sci. Fisheries*, 26: 1132.

Helfrich, P. and A. H. Banner 1968 'Ciguatera fish poisoning. II. General patterns of development in the Pacific.' *Occasional Papers, Bernice P. Bishop Museum*, 23: 371.

Helfrich, P., T. Piyakarnchana and P. S. Miles 1968 'Ciguatera fish poisoning. I. The ecology of ciguateric reef fishes in the Line Islands.' *Occasional Papers, Bernice P. Bishop Museum*, 23: 305.

Irie, T., M. Suzuki and Y. Hayakawa 1969 'Isolation of aplysin, debromoaplysin, and aplysinol from *Laurencia okamurai* Yamada.' *Bull. Chem. Soc. Japan*, 42: 843.

Malo, D. 1951 *'Hawaiian Antiquities.'* 2nd Ed., p. 201. Bernice P. Bishop Museum Spec. Publ. 2: Honolulu.

Matsuda, H., Y. Tomiie, S. Yamamura and Y. Hirata 1967 'The structure of aplysin-20 *Chem. Commun.*: 898.

Moore, R. E. and D. J. Scheuer 1971 'Palytoxin: A new marine toxin from a coelenterate.' *Science*, 172: 495.

Mosher, H. S., F. A. Fuhrman, H. D. Buchwald and H. G. Fischer 1964 'Tarichatoxintetrodotoxin: A potent neurotoxin.' *Science*, 144: 1100.

Nigrelli, R. F. and S. Jakowska 1960 'Efects of holothurin. A steroid saponin from the Bahamian Sea Cucumber *(Actinopyga agassizi)* on various biological systems.' *Ann. N. Y. Acad. Sci.*, 90: 884.

Roller, P., C. Djerassi, R. Cloetens and B. Tursch 1969 'Terpenoids. LXIV. Chemical studies of marine invertebrates. V. The isolation of three new holothurinogenins and their chemical correlation with lanosterol.' *J. Amer. Chem. Soc.*, **91**: 4918.

Rüdiger, W. 1967 'Uber die Abwehrfarbstoffe von Aplysia-Arten. II. Die Struktur von Aplysiaviolin.' *Hoppe-Seyler's Z. Physiol. Chem.*, **348**: 1554.

Shimada, S. 1969 'Antifungal steroid glycoside from Sea Cucumber.' *Science*, **163**: 1462.

Tsuda, K. 1966 'Über Tetrodotoxin, Giftstoff der Bowlfische.' *Naturwissenschaften*, **53**: 171.

Tursch, B., R. Cloetens and C. Djerassi 1970 'Chemical studies of marine invertebrates. VI. Terpenoids. LXV. Praslinogenin, A new holothurinogenin from the Indian Ocean Sea Cucumber *Bohadschia koellikeri.*' *Tetrahedron Letters:* 467.

Tursch, B., I. S. de Souza Guimaraes, B. Gilbert, R. T. Aplin, A. M. Duffield and C. Djerassi 1967 'Chemical studies of marine invertebrates. II. Terpenoids. LVIII. Griseogenin, a new triterpenoid sapogenin of the Sea Cucumber *Halodeima grisea* L.' *Tetrahedron*, **23**: 761.

Watson, M. 1969 'Some aspects of the pharmacology, chemistry and biology of the midgut gland toxins of some Hawaiian Sea Hares, especially *Dolabella auricularia* and *Aplysia pulmonica.*' Ph. D. Dissertation, University of Hawaii.

Winkler, L. R., B. E. Tilton and M. G. Hardinge 1962 'A cholinergic agent from Sea Hares.' *Arch. Int. Pharmacodyn. Therap.*, **137**: 76.

Woodward, R. B. 1964 'The structure of tetrodotoxin.' *Pure Appl. Chem.*, **9**: 49.

Yamada, K., H. Yazawa, M. Toda and Y. Hirata 1968 'The synthesis of (±)-Aplysin and (±)-Debromoaplysin.' *Chem. Commun.*: 1432.

Yamamura, S. and Y. Hirata 1963 'Structures of aplysin and aplysinol, naturally occurring bromo-compounds.' *Tetrahedron*, **19**: 1485.

Yasumoto, T. and Y. Hashimoto 1965 'Properties and sugar compounds of asterosaponin A from Star Fish.' *Agr. Biol. Chem. (Tokyo)*, **29**: 804.

Yasumoto, T. and Y. Hashimoto 1967 'Properties of asterosaponin B isolated from a Star Fish *Asterias amurensis.*' *Agr. Biol. Chem. (Tokyo)*, **31**: 368.

Yasumoto, T., M. Tanaka and Y. Hashimoto 1966 'Distribution of saponin in echinoderms.' *Bull. Jap. Soc. Sci. Fisheries*, **32**: 673.

ISOLATION AND PURIFICATION OF
GYMNODINIUM BREVE TOXIN*

N. M. TRIEFF, J. J. SPIKES, S. M. RAY
and J. B. NASH

*Department of Preventive Medicine and Community Health, and
Department of Pharmacology and Toxicology, University of
Texas Medical Branch, Galveston, and Marine Laboratory,
Texas A & M University, Galveston, Texas U.S.A.*

INTRODUCTION

VARIOUS SPECIES of marine dinoflagellates of genera *Gonyaulax, Gymnodinium, Procentrum*, and others have been found to be causative agents of shellfish poisoning and of mass mortalities of marine animals. Thus, *Gonyaulax catenella* and *Gonyaulax tamarensis* have been found by Sommer *et al.* (1937) to be the source of toxins in shellfish. Various workers have shown *Gonyaulax monilata* to be toxic to fish and the probable cause of fish kills associated with blooms of this dinoflagellate in the Gulf of Mexico (Connell and Cross, 1950; Howell, 1953; and Gates and Wilson, 1960).

The dinoflagellate, *Gymnodinium breve* has been associated with various fish kills in the Gulf of Mexico (Gunter *et al.,* 1948; Wilson and Ray, 1956); it has been suggested as a cause of shellfish poisoning by McFarren *et al.* (1965). Laboratory experiments by Ray and Aldrich (1965, 1967) with *G. breve* have shown that shellfish, feeding on this organism, can poison chicks.

Various investigators have effected an isolation, purification, and partial characterization of some of these marine toxins. Thus, Schantz *et al.* (1957, 1961, 1966, 1967), have clearly demonstrated that the potent toxins which are extracted from clam and mussel tissues and purified are identical to each

*Supported by U.S.P.H.S. FD-00151, NIH ISO 5427 (08), NSF Sea Grant Program (TAMU), and The Robert A. Welch Foundation, H-416.

other as well as to the paralytic poison of *Gonyaulax catenella*. From elemental analysis and physico-chemical measurements, it was found to be an acid-soluble unsaturated nitrogenous base (Schantz, 1969) and a structural formula for *G. catenella* toxin was proposed by Rapoport *et al.* (1964). The structure of *G. catenella* toxin has been elucidated more completely than any other dinoflagellate toxin.

The object of this study was the purification and chemical characterization of the toxin from *G. breve*. Spikes *et al.* (1968) have succeeded in culturing *G. breve*; they have developed an ether extraction method for the toxin and utilized the LD_{50} in mice for evaluating the toxicity of the cultures. A thin-layer chromatographic method of purification of *G. breve* toxin has been developed by Spikes (1971), who has also delineated the pharmacological actions of this toxin (Spikes *et al.*, 1969). These include cardio-vascular changes, some of which are mediated through the autonomic nervous system; the neuromuscular effects included blockade of transmission and later blockade of nerve conduction. No anti-cholinesterase activity was found in this toxin. Other investigators (Martin and Chatterjee, 1969; Paster and Abbott, 1969; Stevens *et al.*, 1968) have also succeeded in concentrating the toxins from *G. breve*, and their results will be examined in more detail in the discussion portion of this paper.

MATERIALS AND METHODS

Growth of *G. breve* cultures

Unialgal cultures of *G. breve* were grown in the artificial seawater media, NH-15 developed by Wilson (Gates and Wilson, 1960). The procedures of culturing, enumeration and extraction generally follow those of Spikes *et al.* (1968).

Extraction of toxin

Prior to extraction, each harvest was adjusted to pH 5.5 with 1.0 N HCl and extracted with diethyl ether in proportions of 150 ml per liter of culture. This procedure produced complete lysis of the cells. The ether was then evaporated to dryness in a mild stream of air or natural gas to yield a tarry

TABLE 1   Stationary phases, solvent systems, and Rf range of toxic fractions for TLC of *Gymnodinium breve* toxin**

Number of Migration	Stationary Phase	Solvent System*	Rf of Toxic Fractions
First	SilicAR/TLC−4GF	Benzene, Ethyl, acetate, Ethanol (absolute), Acetic acid (79:10:10:1)	0.41−0.49
Second	SilicAR/TLC−7GF	Benzene, Ethyl acetate, Ethanol (absolute) (80:10:10)	0.23−0.27
Third	SilicAR/TLC−7GF	Benzene, Ethyl acetate, Secondary Butanol (80:10:10)	0.69

*In percent volume
**Abstracted from Spikes (1971)

black substance with a fish liver odor. The material was dissolved in acetone and after centrifugation the supernatant acetone layer was removed carefully from any non-toxic residue with a capillary pipet. The solution was evaporated and the residue was dissolved in ether for purification by thin-layer chromatography (TLC).

Thin layer chromatographic purification

Standard TLC techniques were used. The detailed procedure can be found in the thesis of Spikes (1971).

Developing media were based on those recommended by Kirchner (1967) for lipids and modified somewhat in order to effect better TLC separations. The developing solvents and the particular TLC plates used are given in Table 1.

In the case of the first migration, approximately 12 separate bands could be visualized under UV light, but this varied depending on the lot of crude toxin and the energy of the UV light. The bands were seen in roughly three groups: (1) several bands of Rf 0.80−0.85 which fluoresced bright red under UV, (2) several bands of subdued red fluorescence of Rf 0.50−0.56, and (3) several bands of subdued blue-green fluorescence or no fluorescence of Rf 0.41−0.49. When the band groups were eluted with ether and bioassayed in mice by the method described below, only the first group (Rf 0.41–0.49) was found to be toxic, and this group of bands was scraped, eluted with ether and prepared for the second migration.

In the second migration, five band groups were visualized under UV: (1) a group at the solvent front, (2) a band group of Rf 0.78–0.82, (3) a band group with Rf 0.31–0.35, (4) a group with Rf 0.23–0.27, (5) a band of non-migrating material at the site of application. The toxin was found in the band Rf 0.23–0.27.

The third migration resulted in little further purification. Aside from the solvent front, there was a discrete green band at Rf 0.82 and a discrete pale green band at Rf 0.69. Only the band at Rf 0.69 contained toxin. Nevertheless, the LD$_{50}$'s of the toxic components from the second and third migrations were found to be virtually identical. In early studies, three TLC migrations were performed, but in later studies, in order to conserve material, only the first two TLC migrations were performed. The purified material was a yellow-green oil.

Column Chromatographic purification

A modification of the method of Martin and Chatterjee (1969) was used for the purification of *G. breve* toxin by column chromatography. A chloroform extract of acidified *G. breve* culture was used as the starting product rather than a chloroform extract of acidified sea water. The same proportions were used as in the ether extraction already described. The chloroform was evaporated with a stream of air and any residual water removed over CaSO$_4$. Sufficient chloroform was added to the dried oil to attain a concentration of about 5 mg/ml. A maximum weight of about 25–30 mg of toxin was employed. The chromatographic column was 1 × 50 cm and contained a 35 cm bed of untreated silica gel, gas chromatographic grade, Davison grade 08 (60/80 mesh). The sample was added to the column, washed with 100 ml of methylene chloride, followed by 100 ml of 95% ethanol for elution. Ten ml fractions were collected from the time when the sample was added. In the chromatographic separation, during the methylene chloride wash, a band appeared which fluoresced red under UV and migrated rapidly down the column to collect in the third and fourth fractions. Only fractions 11–13, which represented the start of the ethanol elution, were toxic. The toxic fractions were combined, dried and weighed (5 mg), dissolved in 5 ml ether and stirred with 1 g of Darco activated charcoal in the cold for 30 minutes.

The cold suspension was filtered and the paper and charcoal washed with ice-cold ether. The filtrate was evaporated to dryness and the residue weighed and tested in mice.

Toxicity studies

The potency of the *G. breve* toxin at each stage of purification was monitored by a bio-assay in mice. In some instances it was necessary to perform only a crude toxicity determination in order to ascertain which TLC band or column fraction was toxic. For each toxic fraction an LD_{50} was determined.

The vehicle used for injection was 0.5% polysorbate 80 in isotonic saline. In order to obtain the solutions for injection, either the ether effluent of the scraped band of the TLC plate or the particular column fraction was evaporated to dryness, dessicated, and weighed in a previously weighed container. About 1 ml of ether was then added to the sample, one drop of polysorbate 80 added, the suspension stirred for several minutes and the ether evaporated. Ten ml of isotonic saline was then added. Various dilutions could then be made with 0.5% polysorbate 80 in isotonic saline.

Intraperitoneal injections of 0.5–1.0 ml were made into white male mice, Swiss strain, of 25–30 g weight. Any mouse dying within 24 hours was counted as a mortality. For the identification of a toxic band, in general, a minimum of 3–4 mice were used.

For the determination of an exact LD_{50} the method of probit transformation of Miller and Tainter (1944) was used. Five dose levels were employed for each stage of purification and at each dosage 10 mice were utilized.

Physico-chemical measurements

Elemental analyses   Elemental Analyses—C, H, O, N, S, P—were performed by Schwarzkopf Microanalytical Laboratory (Woodside, N.Y. 11377).

Molecular weight   The molecular weight determination of TLC purified *G. breve* toxin was performed by Schwarzkopf Microanalytical Laboratory using an osmometric technique with chloroform as the solvent.

Ultra-violet and visible spectral measurements   UV and visible spectral measurements were obtained on a Beckman DB spectrophotometer using tungsten and hydrogen lamps and a 1 cm cell. Various stages of TLC purified *G. breve* were examined in various solvents. The particular solvent always served as the reference solution. In most instances, the absolute concentration of toxin was not known, but dilution was made until a suitable percent transmission was obtained.

Infra-red spectral measurements   IR spectra of purified *G. breve* were determined on the Perkin-Elmer 337 Infra-Red Spectrometer (courtesy of Dr Leland Smith, Department of Biochemistry, University of Texas Medical Branch). Spectra were determined on solutions in carbon tetrachloride and carbon disulfide as well as on KBr pellets containing the toxin.

Mass spectral measurements   Two low resolution mass spectra were run on the TLC purified *G. breve* toxin by Dr Conrad Cone, Department of Chemistry, University of Texas, Austin, Texas. For the first spectrum, the ion source temperature was 105° C with no additional heat on the direct probe, while for the second the ion source was again at 105° C, but the direct probe was also heated.

Optical rotatory measurements   Optical rotatory measurements were obtained on TLC purified toxin in ethanol using a Franz Schmidt and Haensch polarimeter with a 2 decimeter optical tube of 2 ml capacity. The measurements were made using the sodium D line (589 mμ) at 25 ± 2° C. The instrument was set to zero with ethanol in the optical tube.

RESULTS

Thin layer chromatographic purification

Some samples of TLC plates from the first migration are shown in Figures 1 and 2. Figure 1 is a black and white photograph taken under UV light. It may be observed that there is no Rf 0.50–0.56 band group. Essentially no separation has taken place between the Rf 0.41–0.49 (toxic) band group and the Rf 0.50–0.56 band group (subdued red fluorescence). In Figure 2, (a black and white photograph taken under visible light), however, the Rf 0.50–0.56 band group is evident. This variation in migratory behavior in the first migration may be due to differences in composition of the ether extract

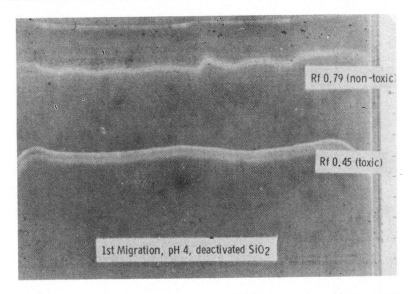

FIGURE 1.   TLC Plate: First migration of *G. breve* toxin, pH 4, deactivated silica. Photograph taken under UV light. Sample inoculated on line flush with bottom of title box on picture

of various *G. breve* lots, and/or slight differences in the activation of the silica gel. Injection into mice indicated that most of the toxicity in the Rf 0.41–0.49 composite band group appears to reside in the Rf 0.41 portion of this band group.

Toxicity studies

The percentage yields for toxicity during the TLC purification process as determined by Spikes (1971) are: first migration–90%; second migration–82%; third migration–55%. Each of these yields is a relative yield showing percentage retention of toxicity, starting from the crude toxin and ending with the indicated step.

The LD_{50} determinations were made on materials obtained from each step in the purification of a single batch of toxin. Spikes (1971) found for the crude ether extract, before acetone treatment, an LD_{50} of 2.2 mg/kg; for the first migration material, 1 mg/kg; and for the second and third migration materials, 0.5 mg/kg. This indicated for the toxin a 2-fold purification by the first TLC migration and a 4–5 fold purification by the second TLC

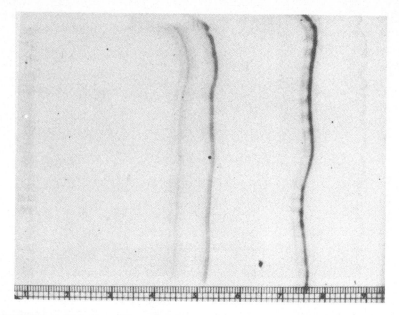

FIGURE 2.   TLC Plate: First migration of *G. breve* toxin, pH 4, deactivated silica. Photograph taken under visible light

migration. A significant batch-to-batch variation in the potency of the crude extract has been found; the LD_{50} on several batches studied has varied from about 2 to 6 mg/kg.

Comparison of ether extraction and TLC purification with chloroform extraction and column chromatographic purification

A single batch of *G. breve* culture was divided into two equal portions of 2.13 $\times$ 10^8 organisms each. One acidified portion extracted with ether yielded 53.2 mg of crude toxin with an LD_{50} of 5.6 mg/kg. The other acidified portion extracted with chloroform yielded 223 mg of crude toxin with an LD_{50} of 19.3 mg/kg. The ether extraction technique, therefore, provided a starting material which is some 3–4 times more concentrated than is obtained by the chloroform extraction. The yield (in mg) divided by the LD_{50} (in mg/kg) gives a measure of the total toxicity. Here, the crude ether extract has a total toxicity of $\dfrac{53.2 \text{ mg}}{5.6 \text{ mg/kg}}$ or 9.5 kg, while the crude chloroform extract has

a total toxicity of $\dfrac{223 \text{ mg}}{19.3 \text{ mg/kg}}$ or 11.5 kg. The unit kg implies that the

particular weight of material in mg can kill one-half of the indicated weight of mice in kg. Thus, the total units of toxicity of the crude chloroform extract are comparable to that of the crude ether extract, at least in the case of one batch of *G. breve*.

With regard to the *G. breve* toxin purified by the method of Martin and Chatterjee (1969), no exact LD_{50} has yet been obtained by us because of insufficient material purified by this technique. However, the toxin purified by this column chromatographic technique is approximately one-tenth as potent as that purified by TLC.

Physico-chemical measurements

Elemental analysis, molecular weight and empirical and molecular formulae The elemental analysis obtained in our TLC purified material (third migration) as well as the elemental analysis listed in the paper by Martin and Chatterjee (1969) for their purified substance II are given in Table 2.

The experimental molecular weight (in $CHCl_3$) and values, derived from the analytical data of Table 2, are listed in Table 3. Their calculation using basic principles of chemistry is fairly obvious and will not be discussed.

Ultra-violet and visible spectra Figures 3, 4 and 5 show the UV-visible spectra for *G. breve* toxin at various stages of purification, in various solvents and at various dilutions. Except for solvent shifts, all spectra at proper dilution show absorption maxima between 275 and 280 mμ. In the case of hexane as solvent, which has no interfering solvent absorption band, a peak is also present at 255 mμ. A more recent quantitative experiment using heptane as solvent and a concentration of 0.05 mg per ml of purified *G. breve* toxin (second TLC migration) showed absorption maxima at 256 mμ and 273 mμ with absorbances of 0.58 and 0.50 respectively. Using our experimental molecular weight of 468, the concentration is equal to 1.07×10^{-4} M, and the calculated molar extinction coefficients (absorptivities) are 5410 and 4670 at 256 mμ and 273 mμ, respectively. The slight absorption maxima in the visible region at about 440 mμ and 510–530 mμ may be due to impurities

TABLE 2   *G. breve* Toxin: elemental analysis*

Elements	Purified Toxin** (method of Spikes *et al.*, 1968)		Martin and Chatterjee (1969) (Substance II)
	Sample 1	Sample 2	
C	63.15	66.81	69.6
H	8.99	9.97	10.49
O	26.36		17.60
N	0.0		0.0
P	1.22		2.0
S	0.0		0.0
Total	99.72		99.69

*Expressed in percent
**Schwartzkopf Microanalytical Laboratory, Woodside, N.Y.

TABLE 3   *G. breve* toxin: molecular weight, empirical and molecular formulae

	Purified Toxin	Martin and Chatterjee (1969) (Substance II)
Experimental Molecular Weight ($CHCl_3$)	468*	650
Calculated Empirical Formula (on the basis of one P/mole	$C_{134}H_{226}O_{49}P$	$C_{90}H_{161}O_{17}P$
Calculated Empirical Weight	2538	1546
Calculated Molecular Formula	$C_{25}H_{42}O_8P_{0.2}$	$C_{38}H_{68}O_7P_{0.4}$
Calculated Molecular Weight	477	649
$\dfrac{\text{Calculated Empirical Weight}}{\text{Experimental Molecular Weight}}$	5.42	2.38

*Osmometric Method (Schwartzkopf Microanalytical Laboratory, Woodside, N.Y.)

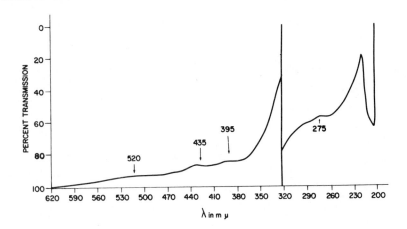

FIGURE 3.   Ultra-violet and visible spectra of crude *G. breve* toxin in ether *vs.* ether reference

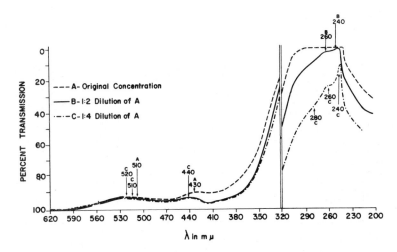

FIGURE 4.   Ultra-violet and visible spectra of *G. breve* toxin purified by TLC (after 3rd migration) in chloroform *vs* chloroform reference

since in some preparations, these peaks were hardly evident.

Infra-red spectra   In Figure 6 are shown the IR spectra of purified *G. breve* toxin in carbon tetrachloride and that of carbon tetrachloride, each versus air. Peaks are evident at 2920 cm^{-1} (3.44 μ), 1725 cm^{-1} (5.80 μ), 1520 cm^{-1}

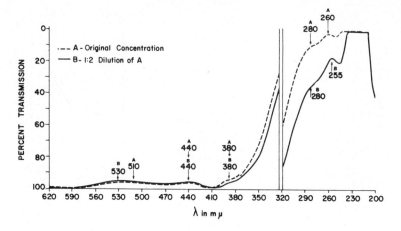

FIGURE 5.   Ultra-violet and visible spectra of *G. breve* toxin purified by TLC (after 3rd migration) in hexane *vs* hexane reference

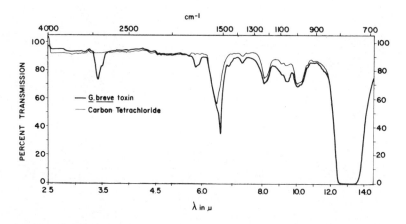

FIGURE 6.   IR spectra of purified *G. breve* toxin in carbon tetrachloride and of carbon tetrachloride *vs* air (% transmission plotted *vs* frequency in cm^{-1} and wavelength in μ)

(0.60 μ), and 1065 cm^{-1} (9.40 μ). No exact measurement of molar extinction coefficients was made.

TABLE 4   Toxicological properties of various *G. breve* toxin preparations

	This Paper	Martin and Chatterjee (1969) (Substance II)	Stevens *et al.* (1968)
LD$_{50}$	0.5 mg/kg*	No data	(A) 13 mg/kg (B) 26 mg/kg
ET$_{50}$	less than 20 min.		(A) 40 min. (B) 146 min.**
Anti-cholinesterase activity	No	Yes	No data
Toxicity to *Fundulus similis* (Striped killifish)	No data	Yes	No data
Stability*	Stable at 100° C for 60 min.; stable for 30+ days at 4° C	No data	No data

*in 0.5% polysorbate 80−saline
**in cottonseed oil

Optical rotatory measurements   A sample of purified *G. breve* toxin at a concentration of 11 mg/25 ml ethanol gave a rotation of +0.08° relative to absolute ethanol, while toxin at a concentration of 2 mg/ml gave an apparent rotation of −0.14°, the negative sign indicating a levo-rotation and the positive sign a dextro-rotation. Both rotations are, within the limits of error of the particular polarimeter used, equal to zero. It is likely that the material is optically inactive and the values of rotation observed are merely a reflection of experimental errors.

Mass spectral measurements   The low resolution mass spectral measurements showed only that the sample was too impure to make any meaningful conclusions from mass spectral data. The only definitive information was a spectral pattern suggesting the presence of dibutyl phthalate, a common plasticizer, which had probably crept into our final product from early processing that made use of some plastic material. Only glass and stainless steel containers will be used in future phases of this work.

TABLE 5   Physico-chemical parameters of *G. breve* toxin preparations

	This Paper	Martin and Chatterjee (1969) (Substance II)
Soluble in	Diethyl ether, chloroform, ethyl alcohol, carbon tetrachloride	Chloroform, ethyl alcohol, carbon tetrachloride
IR Absorption Maxima*	3.44, 5.79, 6.60, 9.4μ	No data given
Functional Groups	Carbonyl	See below
$[\alpha]_D^{25}$	$0°$	$+68°$
Color	Pale yellow	Pale yellow
UV Absorption Maxima, ϵ_M	λ_{max} :256, 273 mμ (heptane) ϵ_M:5410, 4670	No data given
UV Fluorescence	None	No data given
Mass-Spectra**	No fragments identified except for impurity-dibutyl phthalate	No data given but authors state major fragment is $OP(OCH=CH_2)(OCH_2CH=CH_2)$ on the basis of mass spectral and NMR data.
Nuclear Magnetic Resonance	No data	

*Courtesy of Dr Leland Smith, Department of Biochemistry, University of Texas Medical Branch, Galveston, Texas 77550
**Courtesy of Dr Conrad Cone, Department of Chemistry, University of Texas, Austin, Texas

DISCUSSION

Toxicological properties

From our toxicological studies and those of Martin and Chatterjee (1969) it is uncertain whether or not our purified toxin is the same as their substance II (Table 4). They reported only few data in their short paper. They suggest that substance II possesses anti-cholinesterase activity, whereas our toxin does not appear to have any anti-cholinesterase activity (Spikes *et al.*, 1969). Substance I of Martin and Chatterjee (1969), a substance found in the bubbles of the interface between the chloroform and aqueous layers in the extraction procedure, appears to be a proteinaceous cellular debris. We have, however, not yet investigated this substance.

Stevens *et al.* (1968) have recently reported a method for the separation of two toxic components from cultures of *G. breve*. The method involves continuous large-scale liquid-liquid ether extraction of *G. breve* culture followed by a combination of column and thin-layer chromatography using a chloroform-methanol solvent system. Two well separated toxin fractions (to mice) were obtained. The mouse bioassay method of McFarren *et al.* (1965) showed that these two fractions had different LD_{50}'s and that the median effective survival times (ET_{50}), for mice injected with the LD_{50} dose of each toxin, were different. Their data are incorporated into Table 4. It is noteworthy that their extensive extraction procedure produced a material with a higher LD_{50} than the procedure of Spikes *et al.* (1969).

It is difficult to convert the data of Stevens et al. (1968) in a cottonseed oil vehicle to our preparation in a polysorbate 80 vehicle. The latter is known to permit a faster rate of absorption of the toxin than does cottonseed oil. At the LD_{50} dose, our mice generally die in less than 20 minutes, although on occasion a mouse may survive for several hours. No definite conclusion can be made at this stage as to whether our purified toxin consists of a mixture of toxins or a single one; also, if it is a single toxin no conclusion can be made as to whether or not it corresponds to the slow-acting or fast-acting toxin of Stevens *et al.* (1968) until the same lot of purified toxin is compared in cottonseed oil and in polysorbate 80 vehicles. It is noteworthy from the data in Table 4 that the LD_{50} for our purified toxin was approximately 25 times (and our crude toxin was 2 to 6 times) more potent than the fast-acting toxin of Stevens *et al.* (1968). Some of this difference may be attributable to the different vehicles used.

A recent report of Paster and Abbott (1969) shows a hemolytic effect *in vitro* by a toxin extracted from *G. breve* cells by a 2:1 (v/v) chloroformethanol mixture. No *in vivo* studies have been made by these authors. Using the technique of Paster and Abbott, we have found no hemolytic activity to be present in our ether-extracted, TLC-purified toxin.

Physico-chemical properties

The physico-chemical characteristics for our purified toxin and those listed by Martin and Chatterjee (1969) for their substance II are given in Table 5.

As noted in the results section, the elemental analysis is similar but certainly not identical (Table 3). Both toxins, however, contain a small but noteworthy amount of phosphorus. The molecular weights are of the same magnitude, but decidedly different. The calculated empirical and molecular formulae are, again, similar but within such a range that we cannot decide whether the toxins or the degrees of purity are different. Interestingly, for our toxin as well as for the material prepared by Martin and Chatterjee (1969) the empirical formula based on one P/mole gives an empirical weight substantially greater than the experimental molecular weight. This means either that phosphorus is an impurity in the original toxin or that the original *G. breve* toxin fragments either during the processing or during molecular weight determination in chloroform. This ratio of empirical weight to experimental molecular weight was substantially different for our toxin (5.42) than it was for that of Martin and Chatterjee (2.38).

The UV and IR spectra suggest the possibility of certain functional groups being present in the purified toxin. With regard to the UV spectra first, our experimental values are λ_{max} = 256 mμ, ϵ_M = 5410 and λ_{max} = 273 mμ, ϵ_M = 4670 with cut-off at 235 mμ. Absorption maxima with much lower molar extinctions occur at about 440 and 530 mμ. Bauman (1962) lists certain chromophores and auxochromes with their approximate λ_{max} and extinction coefficient values. Some possible structures which might account for the experimental UV spectra are bicyclic aromatic ring structure, aromatic quinone structure, or possibly even dibutyl phthalate.

TABLE 6   IR Absorption maxima and possible contributory functional groups with their characteristic group frequencies

Absorption Maxima		Possible Contributory Functional Groups	Approximate Frequency Range in cm^{-1}
cm^{-1}	μ		
2920	3.44	aliphatic CH_2 —stretching	2850—3000
1725	5.80	carbonyl: aldehyde, ketone or ester	1700—1750
1520	6.60	aliphatic CH_2 —scissors	1400—1500+
1065	9.40	carbonyl	1000—1150

The IR spectral absorption maxima (Figure 6) are listed in Table 6 along with possible contributing functional groups and their characteristic requirements as noted by Szymanski (1964).

The IR spectra thus suggest the presence of a carbonyl functional group. The most definite indication of this is the 1725 cm^{-1} absorption peak. It is likely that the carbonyl compound is aliphatic, although the presence of aromatic groups cannot be completely ruled out.

An alkyl phosphate functional group is also a possibility as shown by a spectrum on a KBr plate (not shown here) in which there were absorption bands between 1000–1100 and 1200–1300 cm^{-1}.

The UV spectra may suggest such structures as a bicyclic aromatic or a quinoid ring, but other chromophores and auxochromes are entirely possible. The present evidence is insufficient to draw definite conclusions.

Our purified material showed no evidence of being optically rotatory. We are, therefore, either dealing with a different toxin than are Martin and Chatterjee (1969) who have observed a fairly high specific rotation, or else the same toxin at different stages of purification in the two laboratories. We may speculate that the red pigment which separates out during the TLC and column chromatography may be a phychoerythrin or similar pigment with a structure similar to chlorophyll, which does have a marked specific rotation (West and Todd, 1956). It is possible that the optical rotation observed by Martin and Chatterjee (1969) may be a result of contamination by this pigment.

CONCLUSIONS

A toxin from the dinoflagellate, *Gymnodinium breve* has been purified and partially characterized by physico-chemical and bioassay studies. The isolation procedure consisted of ether extractions of acidified cultures of *G. breve*, concentration, solution in acetone and successive migrations on TLC plates, pH 4 (first migration) or pH 7 (second and third migrations) with the solvent system consisting of mixtures of benzene, ethylacetate, ethanol (or sec. butanol). The toxin was emulsified in 0.5% polysorbate 80-isotonic saline for the mouse bioassay. The LD_{50} of the crude toxin in mice by the intraperitoneal route was about 2.2 mg/kg and that of the material isolated from the second and third migrations was about 0.5 mg/kg showing about a four-fold purification. Elemental analysis of the purified material indicated the following percent composition: C (63.15), H (8.99), P (1.22), and O (26.36). The molecular weight obtained was 468, so that the calculated 'molecular' formula was $C_{25}H_{42}O_8P_{0.2}$, showing either that phosphorus was an impurity or that fragmentation of the molecule had occurred. Infra-red spectra revealed an aliphatic carbonyl compound. The purified material is not optically active and possesses certain chromophore groups in the ultra-violet range. It is highly stable and possesses no anti-cholinesterase activity. The properties of our toxin were compared with those of Martin and Chatterjee and Stevens *et al.*

ACKNOWLEDGMENTS

This work was supported by grants from the USPHS, NIH, the NSF Sea Grant Program and the Robert A. Welch Foundation. We gratefully acknowledge the assistance and advice from the following: Dr Leland Smith, Department of Biochemistry, University of Texas Medical Branch, Galveston, Texas, for help and advice with the interpretation of the infra-red spectra and the purification of the toxin; Dr Conrad Cone, University of Texas, Department of Chemistry, Austin, Texas, for making and interpreting mass spectral determinations on our purified toxin; Dr Sydney Ellis, Department of Pharmacology and Toxicology, University of Texas Medical Branch for suggestions; Mrs Anita Sievers Aldrich, Mr Terrence Eakens and Mr Ray Jones for technical assistance.

SUMMARY

The toxin from the dinoflagellate, *Gymnodinium breve*, previously reported by McFarren *et al.* to cause symptoms of paralytic shellfish poisoning, was isolated by a thin layer chromatographic (TLC) procedure and partially characterized by physico-chemical and toxicological studies. The isolation procedure consisted of ether extraction of acidified cultures of *G. breve*, evaporation of the ether, and successive migrations of the acetone-soluble portion of the residue on TLC silica gel plates. The first migration used a TLC-4GF plate (Mallinckrodt), and a developer of benzene, ethyl acetate, ethanol, acetic acid (49:10:10:1); the toxin appeared in several closely spaced bands with rf 0.41–0.49. In the second migration, a TLC-7GF plate was used with developer of benzene, ethyl acetate, ethanol (80:10:10), the toxic material being eluted with ether from bands with rf 0.23–0.27 with recovery of 80% of the total toxicity. A third migration was performed with TLC-7GF plate and a developer of benzene, ethyl acetate, sec. butanol (80:10:10) but no detectable increase in purification occurred, while appreciable losses in toxicity were found (55–60% total recovery). The effluent from each TLC migration was emulsified in 0.5% polysorbate 80 in saline and the LD_{50} was determined with mice. The LD_{50} of the crude toxin was about 2.2. mg/kg and that of the material eluted from the second migration was 0.5 mg/kg showing roughly a four-fold purification by the TLC procedure. The toxin was also isolated by a column chromatographic procedure based on that of Martin and Chatterjee. The toxin isolated by our TLC procedure has similar characteristics (toxicity, physical and chemical) to substance II of the latter workers. Elemental analysis on the TLC-isolated material revealed the presence of C (63.2%), H (8.9%), P (1.2%) and O (26.4%). A molecular weight of 468 was found by osmometry. Other physico-chemical techniques were also employed for characterization.

References

Bauman, R. P. 1962 'Absorption Spectroscopy.' pp. 316–321. John Wiley and Sons, Inc., New York.

Connell, C. H. and J. B. Cross 1950 'Mass mortality of fish associated with the protozoan Gonyaulax in the Gulf of Mexico.' Science, 112: 359.

Gates, J. A. and W. B. Wilson 1960 'The toxicity of Gonyaulax monilata Howell to Mugil cephalus.' Limnol. Oceanog., 5: 171.

Gunter, G., R. H. Williams, C. C. Davis and F. G. W. Smith 1948 'Catastrophic mass mortality of marine animals and coincident phytoplankton bloom on the west coast of Florida, November 1946 to August 1947.' Ecol. Monographs, 18: 311.

Howell, J. F. 1953 'Gonyaulax monilata sp. nov., the causative dinoflagellates of a red tide on the east coast of Florida in August-September 1951.' Trans. Am. Microscop. Soc., 72: 153.

Kirchner, J. G. 1967 'Thin Layer Chromatography.' Interscience Publishers, New York.

Martin, D. F. and A. B. Chatterjee 1969 'Isolation and characterization of a toxin from the Florida red tide organism.' Nature, 221: 59.

McFarren, E. F., H. Tanabe, F. J. Silva, W. B. Wilson, J. E. Campbell and K. H. Lewis 1965 'The occurrence of a ciguateralike poison in oysters, clams, and Gymnodinium breve cultures.' Toxicon, 3: 111.

Miller, L. C. and M. L. Tainter 1944 'Estimation of the E.D. 50 and its error by means of logarithmic-probit graph paper.' Proc. Soc. Exptl. Biol. Med., 57: 261.

Paster, Z. and B. C. Abbott 1969 'Hemolysis of rabbit erythrocytes by Gymnodinium breve Toxin.' Toxicon, 7: 245.

Rapoport, H., M. D. Brown, R. Oesterlin and W. Schuett 1964 'Saxitoxin.' 147th National Meeting of the American Chemical Society, Philadelphia, Pa.

Ray, S. M. and D. V. Aldrich 1965 'Gymnodinium breve: Induction of shell-fish poisoning in chicks.' Science, 148: 1748.

Ray, S. M. and D. V. Aldrich 1967 'Ecological interactions of toxic dinoflagellates and molluscs in the Gulf of Mexico.' In: Animal Toxins, Russell, F. E. and P. R. Saunders (eds.), p. 75 Pergamon Press, Oxford.

Schantz, E. J., J. D. Mold, D. W. Stanger, J. Shavel, F. J. Riel, J. P. Bowden, J. M. Lynch, R. S. Wyler, B. Riegel and H. Sommer 1957 'Paralytic shellfish poison. VI. A procedure for the isolation and purification of the poison from toxic clam and mussel tissues.' J. Am. Chem. Soc., 79: 5230.

Schantz, E. J., J. D. Mold, W. L. Howard, J. P. Bowden, D. W. Stanger, J. M. Lynch, O. P. Wintersteiner, J. D. Dutcher, D. R. Walters and B. Riegel 1961 'Paralytic Shellfish Poison. VIII. Some chemical and physical properties of purified clam and mussel poisons.' Can. J. Chem., 39: 2117.

Schantz, E. J., J. M. Lynch, G. Vayvada, K. Matsumoto and H. Rapoport 1966 'The purification and characterization of the poison produced by Gonyaulax catenella in Axenic culture.' Biochemistry, 5: 1191.

Schantz, E. J. 1967 'Biochemical studies on purified Gonyaulax catenella poison.' In: Animal Toxins, Russell, F. E. and P. R. Saunders (eds.), p. 91. Pergamon Press Oxford.

Schantz, E. J. 1969 'Studies on shellfish poisons.' Agric. Food Chem., 17: 413.

Sommer, H., W. F. Whedon, C. A. Kofoid and R. Stohler 1937 'Relation of paralytic shellfish poison to certain plankton organisms of the genus Gonyaulax.' Arch. Pathol., 242: 537.

Spikes, J. J., S. M. Ray, D. V. Aldrich and J. B. Nash 1968 'Toxicity variations of *Gymnodinium breve* cultures.' *Toxicon.*, 5: 171.

Spikes, J. J., S. M. Ray and J. B. Nash 1969 'Studies of the pharmacology and toxicology of *Gymnodinium breve* toxin.' *The Pharmacologist*, 11: 283.

Spikes, J. J. 1971 'Extraction, concentration and biologic effects of a toxic material from *Gymnodinium breve.*' Ph.D. Dissertation, University of Texas Medical Branch (Galveston, Texas).

Stevens, A. A., J. M. Cummins and W. F. Hill, Jr 1968 'A method for separation of two toxic components from cultures of *Gymnodinium breve.*' *Gulf Coast Marine Health Sciences Laboratory (Dauphin Island, Alabama 36528), Special Report GCMHSL-68-3.*

Szymanski, H. A. 1964 '*IR–Theory and Practice of Infrared Spectroscopy.*' Plenum Press, New York.

West, E. S. and W. R. Todd 1956 '*Textbook of Biochemistry.*' p. 1029. The Macmillan Company, New York.

Wilson, W. B. and S. M. Ray 1956 'The occurrence of *Gymnodinium breve* in the Western Gulf of Mexico.' *Ecology*, 37: 388.

POISONOUS ALKALOIDS IN THE BODY TISSUES OF THE GARDEN TIGER MOTH *(ARCTIA CAJA* L.) AND THE CINNABAR MOTH *(TYRIA (= CALLIMORPHA) JACOBAEAE* L.) *(LEPIDOPTERA)*

R. T. APLIN

Dyson Perrins Laboratory, University of Oxford, England
and
M. ROTHSCHILD

Ashton, Peterborough, England

Dedication: It is a great privilege to acknowledge our admiration and gratitude to Professor H. Mendelssohn on his sixtieth birthday. He has, in his own quiet, subtle and inimitable way, provided inspiration for zoologists all over the world. We thank him for his help and encouragement.

INTRODUCTION

AT THE 2ND INTERNATIONAL SYMPOSIUM on Animal and Plant Toxins in Israel (Tel-Aviv, 1970) we read a paper in collaboration with T. Reichstein and J. von Euw on Toxic Lepidoptera, a short general account of which is appearing in Toxicon (1971). It was therefore agreed that we should here present a particular section of this paper in greater detail, the work for which was carried out by two of us at Ashton and Oxford, England.

In this investigation we tested *Arctia caja* L. to determine whether, like the related species *Tyria* (= *Callimorpha*) *jacobaeae* L., (Aplin *et al.*, 1968) it was capable of storing the poisonous alkaloids from the food plant *Senecio vulgaris* L. in its body tissues. We also examined further material of both *T. jacobaeae* and *Senecio jacobaea* L.

MATERIALS AND METHODS

We obtained eggs of the garden tiger moth from females caught in a light trap at Ashton, Peterborough and Elsfield, Oxford, and reared the larvae on groundsel (*S. vulgaris*) grown in specific areas in the two gardens. We collected larvae of the cinnabar moth at Weeting Heath, Norfolk and Ashton, Peterborough, feeding on ragwort (*S. jacobaea*) and continued to rear the caterpillars on this plant obtained from the garden at Ashton, samples of which were examined for their alkaloid content. Likewise the cinnabar moths which we fed on groundsel were found in the wild on this species of plant and were reared upon it until pupation. The eggs of the cinnabar were collected on our behalf by Dr John Dempster at Weeting Heath. Unfortunately the eggs of our groundsel-reared *caja* were delayed in the post and hatched before they could be tested. Frass was collected from both species of caterpillar feeding on the two different species of *Senecio*.

The total alkaloids were isolated by partition of the methanol soluble material, which was obtained by maceration of both plant and insect in methanol, between chloroform and 1 N sulphuric acid. The buff coloured aqueous acidic solution was treated with zinc dust to reduce to the free bases any N-oxides which were present. Concentrated ammonia was added to make the solution basic, and this, followed by isolation with chloroform, gave the total alkaloids (Tables 1–5). Analysis by gas-liquid chromatography* (Chalmers *et al.*, 1965) of the total alkaloids which were present in the plants and insects gave the composition shown in Tables 1–3.

Identification of the chief component from each source, with the exception of the imago alkaloids, was confirmed by isolation and comparison of its mass spectrum with that of an authentic sample. The composition agrees well with that described in the literature (Leonard, 1950, 1960; Warren, 1970) for *S. jacobaea*.

---

*On a Pye 104–14 gas chromatograph equipped with a flame ionization detector and a 1 per cent SE 30 on 100–120 mesh Gas Chrom Q column, operating at 175° with an argon carrier gas flow of 35 ml/min.

TABLE 1   Seasonal variation of alkaloids in the groundsel (*Senecio vulgaris*)

	Collecting date			
	14/6/68	19/7/68	20/8/68	5/12/68
	(Garden, Elsfield, Oxford)	(Garden, Ashton, Peterborough)		
Plant, dry weight, g	77	33	10	14
Total % of alkaloid, dry weight	0.23*	0.20	0.28	0.19*
Senecionine, %	10	10	10	10
Seneciphylline, %	65	70	65	60
Integerrimine, %	25	20	25	30

*Very young plants

TABLE 2   Seasonal variation of alkaloids in the ragwort (*Senecio jacobaea*)

	Collecting date (at Ashton)							
	20/5/68	18/6/68	19/7/68		20/8/68		4/10/68	5/12/68
Plant, dry weight, g	21	70	55	44	5	36	35	14
Total % of alkaloids, dry weight	0.33*	0.52	0.40+	0.79†	0.25	0.22†	0.26	0.23*
Senecionine, %	T	T	T	T	T	T	T	T
Seneciphylline, %	10	10	5	45	40	25	40	20
Integerrimine, %	T	5	15	10	10	20	15	10
Jacobine, %	45	50	15	5	T	T	10	45
Jacozine, %	25	25	60	40	40	55	30	20
Jacoline, %	20	10	5	T	5	T	T	5

* Very young plants
+ Zn reduction stage omitted
† Different collecting site (water-garden, 100 yards distant)
T-Trace

TABLE 3   Site variation of alkaloids in the ragwort (*Senecio jacobaea*)

	18/6/68 Ashton Terrace	26/6/68 Weeting Heath	20/8/68· Ashton Terrace	20/8/68 Ashton water-garden
Plant, dry weight, g	70	51	35	14
Total % of alkaloids, dry weight	0.52	0.24	0.25	0.23
Senecionine	Trace	Trace	Trace	Trace
Seneciphylline, %	10	Trace	40	25
Integerrimine, %	5	5	10	20
Jacobine, %	50	40	Trace	Trace
Jacozine, %	25	20	40	55
Jacoline, %	10	30	5	Trace

TABLE 4   Alkaloid concentrations in Lepidoptera fed on groundsel (*S. vulgaris*)

Source	Dry weight, g	Total % of alkaloids, dry weight
Arctia caja (Garden Tiger)		
Imagos Oct. 1969	2.5	1.10
Pupae Sept. 1969	4.5	1.05
Frass	2.0	0.21
Plant Sept./Oct. 1969	–	0.24
Tyria jacobaeae (Cinnabar)		
Pupae	23.6	0.95
Frass	2.0	0.08
Plant	–	0.26
Spodoptera littoralis Imagos	3.4	Absent*
Melanchra persicariae Imagos	1.8	Absent*

*Both by gas liquid chromatography and mass spectrometric analysis

TABLE 5   Alkaloid concentrations in *Tyria jacobaeae* fed on ragwort (*S. jacobaea*)

Source		Dry weight, g	Total % of alkaloids dry weight
Cinnabar pupae	)	3.6	0.73
Cinnabar eggs	) Weeting) Heath) July 1968	0.9 (wet wt.)	Absent*
Frass	)	36	0.09
Plant	)	51	0.24
Frass	) Ashton	37	0.15
Plant	) July 1968	44	0.79

*Both by gas liquid chromatography and mass spectrometric analysis

THE ALKALOID CONTENT OF THE FOOD PLANTS

Nine collections of the groundsel were made from Oxford and Ashton, and all were found to be positive for Senecionine (I), Seneciphylline (II) and Integerrimine (III). Four of these collections were further analysed in order to estimate the total quantity of the alkaloids present and their individual concentrations. These results are set out in Table 1. It will be seen that there is relatively little seasonal variation, the overall percentage (of the dry weight) and the relative concentrations of the three alkaloids remains approximately similar in June, July, August and December. Nor is there any difference between very young plants collected in Oxford in June and Ashton in December.

Eight collections of ragwort were made at Ashton (see Table 2), six from an uncut area of a lawn on a terrace-garden, and two from an uncut lawn in a sunken water-garden. The distance between these two sites was less than 100 yards. Another collection was made at Weeting Heath, Norfolk (abut 200 miles from Ashton) from whence some larvae and eggs of the cinnabar were obtained (Table 5). In contrast to the groundsel, the ragwort exhibits both site and seasonal variation (Table 3) and no doubt variation from year to year would also become apparent if this aspect was investigated. Thus, for example, plants collected in the Ashton water-garden in July contained ten times as much Seneciphylline as those from the terrace lawn. A marked difference was also evident between the samples from Ashton and Weeting

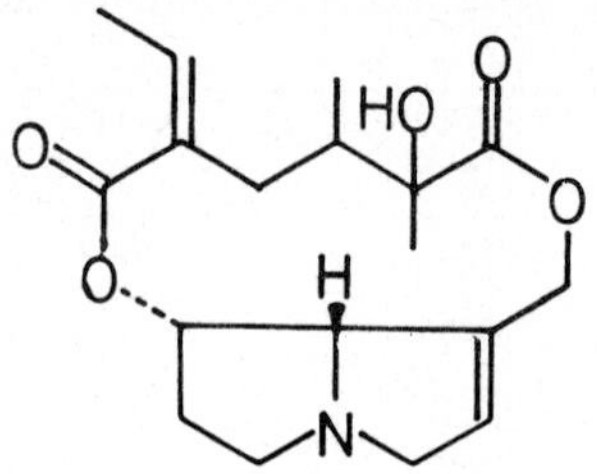

Senecionine   I

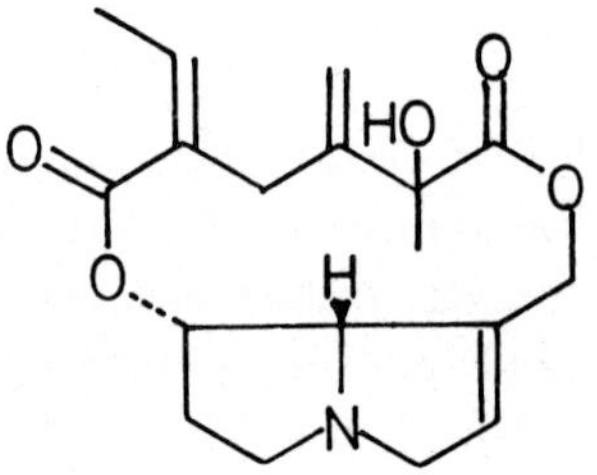

Seneciphylline   II

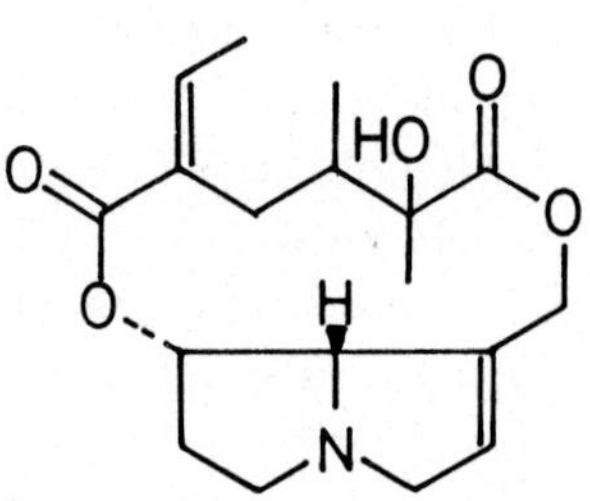

Integerrimine   III

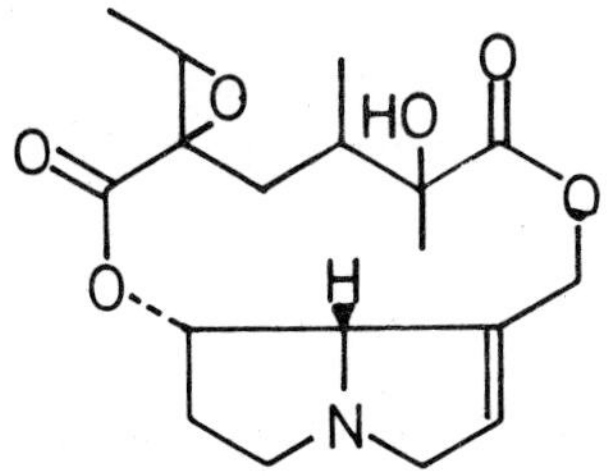

Jacobine   IV

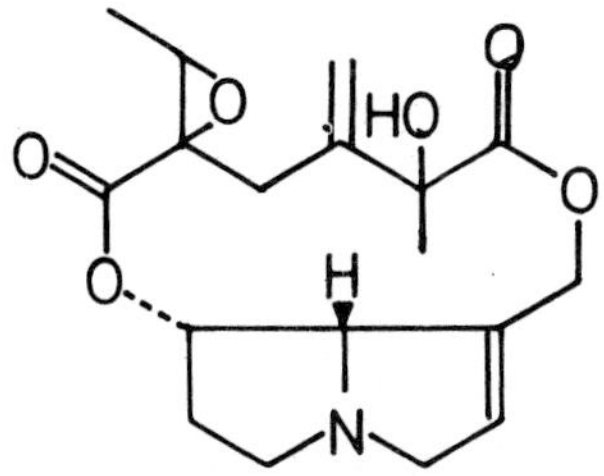

Jacozine   V

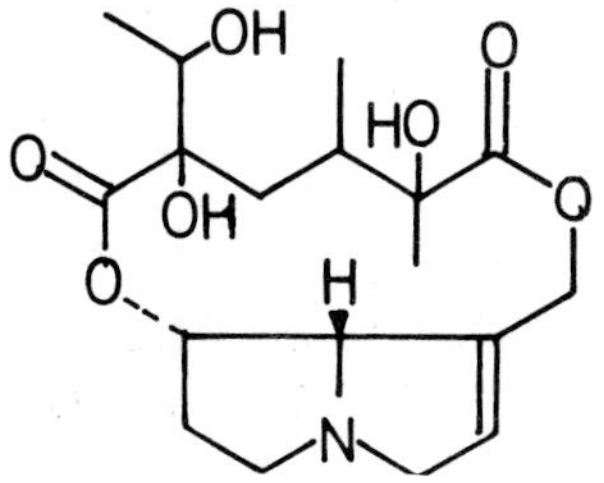

Jacoline   VI

Heath. The relative concentration of Senecionine (I), Seneciphylline (II) and Integerrimine (III) is low in spring and rises as the season advances, whereas Jacobine (IV) and Jacoline (VI) are at high levels in the spring but drop markedly in July and August (Table 2).

Omission of the zinc dust reduction stage in the isolation procedure (Table 2, col. 19/7/68) indicated that Seneciphylline is present mainly as the water soluble N-oxide. The metabolite ($C_{15}H_{23}NO_5$) found in both insects is absent from the food plant.

COMPOSITION OF THE ALKALOIDS PRESENT IN THE BODIES OF GROUNDSEL-FED *A. CAJA* AND *T. JACOBAEAE* AND THE FRASS FROM THEIR LARVAL STAGES

Both the cinnabar and tiger, as pupae and adults, show a very similar distribution of alkaloids in their body tissues which mirrors that found in the groundsel:—

Senecionine	Seneciphylline	Integerrimine	Metabolite ($C_{15}H_{23}NO_5$)
ca 5%	50—60%	23—30%	15—20%

The total percentage of alkaloids (dry weight) is higher in the insect than in the food plant (Table 4). This may be due to an efficient storage system in the insects but could also be the result of fluctuations in the alkaloid concentrations in certain samples of the food plant, despite the fact that they were all collected from the same garden site. In the frass obtained from groundsel-fed larvae of the cinnabar the level of alkaloids relative to the plant was greatly diminished (Table 4) but not in the tiger despite the fact that the latter species was apparently storing them efficiently.

COMPOSITION OF ALKALOIDS PRESENT IN THE BODIES OF RAGWORT-FED *T. JACOBAEAE* AND THE FRASS FROM THEIR LARVAL STAGES

All the six alkaloids (I-VI) from the plant, together with the metabolite (Aplin *et al.*, 1968) were detected in the pupae and adults, but the relative concentrations of the alkaloids had been altered significantly. The Senecionine (I), Seneciphylline (II) and Integerrimine (III) group of alkaloids is dominant in the insect (60—70%) whereas the Jacobine (IV), Jacozine (V)

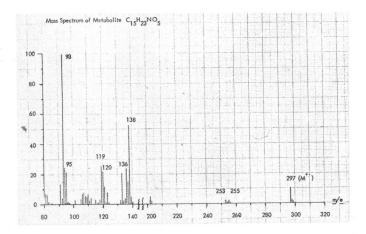

FIGURE 1.   Mass spectrum of Metabolite $C_{15}H_{23}NO_5$

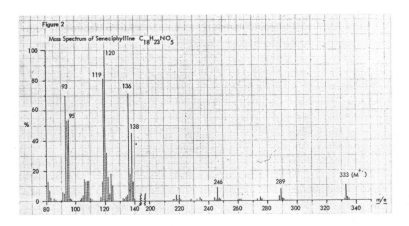

FIGURE 2.   Mass spectrum of Seneciphylline $C_{18}H_{23}NO_5$

and Jacoline (VI) group is dominant in the plant (40–60%). In the frass the total alkaloid concentration was diminished relative to the food plant (Table 5) as in the case of the groundsel-fed cinnabar, but, as might be expected from the analysis of the pupal stage, the relative concentrations of the Senecionine, Seneciphylline and Integerrimine group had dropped by approximately 10% in comparison with the Jacobine, Jacozine and Jacoline group. Thus Seneciphylline is the major alkaloid stored by both species of

TABLE 6   Relative proportions of the alkaloids present in the pupae of *Tyria jacobaeae* and in *Senecio jacobaea*

		Pupae *T. jacobaeae* (Average of two trials)	Plant *S. jacobaea* (Average of Sept. & Oct. samples)	Pupae *T. jacobaeae* & *A. caja*	Plant *S. vulgaris*
Senecionine	)			5	10
Seneciphylline	) %	60–70	40–60	50–60	65–70
Integerrimine	)			23–30	20–30
Jacobine	)				
Jacozine	) %	10–15	40–60		Absent
Jacoline	)				
Metabolite	) %	20–25	Absent	15–20	Absent

moth, although not dominant in the ragwort plants. The eggs of the cinnabar lacked both *Senecio* alkaloids and the metabolite (Table 5).

THE METABOLITE ($C_{15}H_{23}NO_5$)

It is interesting that the metabolite* which we detected previously in the cinnabar (Aplin *et al.*, 1968) is also present in *A. caja* fed on groundsel. On the basis of a comparison of its mass spectrum (Figure 1) with that of Seneciphylline (Figure 2) one can deduce that it has the characteristic fragmentation of the *Senecio* alkaloids (Neuner-Jehle *et al.*, 1965) and appears to contain a modified ester substituent attached to a Retronecine (VII) type nucleus.

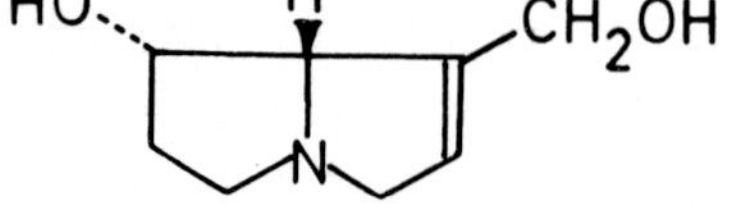

Retronecine   VII

---

*Due to a typing error this formula was erroneously recorded as $C_{15}H_{25}NO_5$ in Nature 1968.

ADDITIONAL OBSERVATIONS

In the wild, groundsel is an alternative food plant for the cinnabar but to our knowledge no observations have been made on the selection by the cinnabar of these two plants.

We noticed that in the early part of the season the ragwort in the garden at Oxford was entirely devoid of cinnabar larvae and we were forced to collect them from groundsel, on which plant they were quite plentiful. Later in the season, when the ragwort was in flower, the selfsame plants were attacked by large numbers of cinnabar larvae, and a few were completely defoliated.

We were sufficiently impressed by the marked preference of the cinnabars for groundsel in the spring in Oxford to compare the seasonal difference in the alkaloid content of this plant. The laying preference of the moth is clearly an aspect of the problem which merits further investigation. Possibly the female was selecting Seneciphylline rich plants on which to oviposit (Table 2) but they may also show a predilection for a food plant growing on bare ground, the advantages of which have been stressed by Dempster (1970) (see below, p. 590).

During the course of these experiments we had numerous opportunities of feeding both *A. caja* and *T. jacobaeae* reared on the same food plant (*S. vulgaris*) to various caged avian predators, both experienced and inexperienced individuals. It was not unexpected to find that in these circumstances *T. jacobaeae* was still a far more repellent insect than *A. caja* (Frazer *et al.*, 1960) and obviously possesses powerful deterrent qualities unconnected with its food plant (Rothschild *et al.*, 1970).

In addition to the two arctiids, two other species of noctuiids, *Spodoptera littoralis* (Boisduval) and *Melanchra persicariae* L. were reared on groundsel and tested for their alkaloid content. They proved not to store these substances in their body tissues. Unfortunately their frass was not collected so it is not known if they excreted the alkaloids unchanged as in the case of *Protoparce sexta* (Johan.) fed on tobacco, or, if, like *Prodenia eridania* Cram., they metabolised these substances (Self *et al.*, 1964). It is interesting nevertheless that the ability to excrete or metabolise the poisonous secondary plant substances is associated with nocturnal habits and cryptic coloration, whereas the ability to store them has, until now, been found only in diurnal or semi diurnal species with aposematic characteristics.

It is worth noting that the eggs of the cinnabar which are bright yellow in colour do not store the *Senecio* alkaloids. It is safe to assume that they contain some other deterrent. The eggs of the Monarch (*D. plexippus*) and the grasshopper (*P. bufonius*) contain cardenolides (von Euw *et al.*, 1967; Reichstein *et al.*, 1968) and the eggs of *Zygaena* contain HCN (Jones *et al.*, 1962), and those of the tiger* a highly toxic substance thought to be a protein (Frazer *et al.*, 1960).

DISCUSSION

The Arctiidae are an unusually interesting group of warningly coloured moths, many of which are diurnal in their habits. The few so far investigated (Rothschild *et al.*, 1970) are known to contain toxic or irritant substances which are secreted by the moths themselves. Almost all of them when disturbed react by aposematic displays (Blest, 1964; Rothschild *et al.*, 1966) associated with offensive secretions (which in some instances can be ejected together with their own haemolymph for considerable distances, e.g. *Apantesis virgo* [L.] [Dethier, 1939]), sound production and repellent scents. The food plants of arctiids are extremely varied and some species are virtually polyphagous although low growing plants are preferred, while others again are restricted to a single genus or a single species. A noteworthy feature of the feeding habits of this group is their predilection for poisonous plants. Thus the larvae of at least nineteen species are recorded feeding on Asclepiadaceae, and five on *Crotalaria***, *A. caja* itself has been known to feed occasionally on laburnum (*Laburnum anagyroides* L.), lily-of-the-valley (*Convallaria majalis* L.), monkshood (*Aconitum napellus* L.), dog's mercury (*Mercurialis perennis* L.), potato (*Solanum tuberosum* L.), foxglove (*Digitalis purpurea* L.), nettle (*Urtica dioica* L.), etc. There are certain very definite advantages which accrue to moths and butterflies which can feed on protected plants. Thus their early stages are preserved from destruction by herbivores; the presence of poisonous, often apparently bitter tasting elements in the gut render them to a certain extent inedible, and they enjoy the advantages conferred by the presence of other aposematic insects in their immediate vicinity. This situation is particularly evident where *Asclepias* are concerned, but also to a lesser extent in the case of other plants such as the

---

*We have since reported the presence of pyrrolizidine alkaloids in the eggs of *Arctia caja* (Aplin & Rothschild 1971 in press).

**One of the species (*Utethesia bella* L.) which feeds on *Crotalaria* secretes the same choline ester in its defensive glands as *A. caja* (Rothschild *et al.*, 1970) and it too can store pyrrolizidine alkaloids.

nettle (Rothschild, 1964). There is also a subtle but very real advantage conferred by the grazing down of grass and other vegetation round poisonous plants (by cattle and other animals) thereby removing from their immediate vicinity the cover required by the predatory arthropods which attack them (Wilkinson, 1965; Dempster, 1970). It is not necessary, therefore, to assume that because arctiids are feeding on poisonous plants they must be able to store such a wide variety of toxins. In fact the only two species of arctiids reared on *Asclepias* which we have so far examined (Rothschild *et al.*, 1970) lacked cardenolides in their body tissues. There is no doubt, however, that both *T. jacobaeae* and *A. caja* store the toxic alkaloids from *Senecio* but their role in these insects' defence mechanism is enigmatical; but this is chiefly because it is difficult to know if the animal which ingests these alkaloids suffers any immediate discomfort. Schoental (personal communication) has observed that following large doses given intragastrically, rats appeared 'unhappy' and some died within 2–3 days from acute liver necrosis. It is difficult to believe that some pain and discomfort is not felt within minutes of ingestion of pyrrolizidine alkaloids. The long term damage to the liver (Schoental and MaGee, 1959; Hill *et al.*, 1960; Mattocks, 1968) is well known, but in order to act as an efficient deterrent linked to warning coloration, the disagreeable effects of swallowing these alkaloids must be more or less immediate. Long delayed effects would not be associated with the prey concerned. Nevertheless the fact that the two aposematic groundsel-fed moths store *Senecio* alkaloids, whereas the two cryptic species we examined do not, suggests that these substances play some part in the moths' defence mechanism.

The variation which we found in the concentration of alkaloids in *S. jacobaea* both in time and space is not surprising. Klásek *et al.* (1968, p. 1089) have also noted seasonal variation in the alkaloids of *Senecio alpinus* (L.) Scop. Any practical farmer or horticulturalist is constantly reminded of the great variation in secondary plant substances, whether it is the essential oils in lavender, the active terpinoids in *Cannabis*, the alkaloids in *Papaver*, the sugar in sugar-beet, the HCN in various cyanogenic strains of clover and vetches, or cardenolides in *Digitalis* grown for medical purposes (Flück in Swain, 1963). Parallel variation can be expected in the secondary plant products stored in the body tissues of insects. Brower (1969) has recently demonstrated that the Monarch (*D. plexippus*) mirrors the concentration of various cardenolides found in different species of *Asclepias* on which it feeds. A similar situation is evident with the alkaloids in the groundsel, but there are also considerable differences in the concentrations found in a single species of *Senecio*, which one can confidently expect will also be reflected in the cinnabar and tiger. In a population of aposematic insects one can expect an overall picture of unpalatability but also widespread variation in the quantity and quality of the poisons stored in the tissues, even in those species confined to one food plant, and this will be apparent not only in different localities (and, as we have seen, such differences can occur in plants growing on two adjacent grass lawns) but at different times of the year and probably from one season to the next. Such a situation must also exert pressure on the species in question to evolve and develop deterrents other than, or in addition to, those derived from the food plant; it is evident that various aposematic insects, the Monarch included, have done so, for they are unacceptable to many avian predators for reasons other than their indigestible qualities.

The Monarch and its allies, once having shifted onto plants of the family Asclepiadaceae (Ehrlich and Raven, 1965) and acquired the toxic cardenolides from the latex, are destined to evolve the warning life-style. Another situation is illustrated by certain species of zygaenids. These aposematic moths secrete substances possessing toxic or irritant properties including HCN to which they themselves are relatively resistant (Jones *et al.*, 1962). Consequently they are able to feed on the cyanogenic strains of clovers and vetches and thereby obtain the additional advantages which accrue to species associated with well protected plants. Possibly the tiger and cinnabar belong to yet another slightly different category—i.e. aposematic insects, already protected by warning colour and their own toxic secretions, which considerably improve their chances of survival by developing the ability to feed on a wide range of poisonous plants.

CONCLUSIONS

These observations show that *A caja* and *T. jacobaeae* reared on the groundsel store *Senecio* alkaloids derived from the food plant in their body tissues. The distribution of these substances in both insects and in the groundsel is rather similar but the concentration is higher in the insect and greatly diminished in the larval frass. A somewhat different situation is apparent if *T. jacobaeae* is reared on *S. jacobaea*. Although the various alkaloids detected in the plant are also found in the moth, their relative concentrations are significantly altered both in the pupa and adult, and also in the larval frass. It appears that the *T.*

jacobaeae is selectively storing Seneciphylline which, in the ragwort (Table 2) is present mainly as the N-oxide.

There is apparently little if any seasonal or regional variation in the samples of *S. vulgaris* so far examined, whereas the concentration of the various alkaloids present in *S. jacobaea* varies considerably both in time and space.

No alkaloids were detected in the eggs of *T. jacobaeae* nor in the adults of two species of cryptic noctuiids reared on *S. vulgaris*.

ACKNOWLEDGMENTS

We wish to express our gratitude to Mr Bob Ford, Dr John Dempster and Dr C. F. Rivers for collecting and breeding material on our behalf. We are also greatly indebted to Professor C. C. J. Culvenor for authentic samples of the alkaloids (I–VI) shown in Tables 1 and 2, Dr John Dempster and Dr Peter Harris for supplying information regarding arthropod predators and Dr A. T. Mattocks and Dr R. Schoental for help and advice.

SUMMARY

Two aposematic moths, *Arctia caja* L. and *Tyria jacobaeae* L. store the poisonous alkaloids derived from their food plants in their body tissues while two cryptic noctuiid moths do not. Seneciphylline is the principal alkaloid stored and the concentration in the insects is higher than in either species of food plant. Variation in the alkaloid concentrations in the ragwort (*Senecio jacobaea* L.) occurs both in time and space.

References

Aplin, R. T., M. H. Benn and M. Rothschild 1968 'Poisonous alkaloids in the body tissues of the Cinnabar Moth (*Callimorpha jacobaeae* L.).' *Nature (London)*, 219: 747.

Aplin, R. T. and M. Rothschild 1971 'Toxins in Tiger Moths (Arctiidae: Lepidoptera).' *In:* 'Pesticide Chemistry', A. Tahori (ed.) (in press).

Blest, A. D. 1964 'Protective display and sound production in some New World arctiid and ctenuchid moths.' *Zoologica, Stuttgart*, 49: 161.

Brower, L. P. 1969 'Ecological Chemistry.' *Sci. Am.*, 220: 22.

Chalmers, A. H., C. C. J. Culvenor and L. W. Smith 1965 'Characterisation of pyrrolizidine alkaloids by gas, thin layer and paper chromatography.' *J. Chromatogr.*, 20: 270.

Dempster, J. P. 1970 'Some effects of grazing on the population ecology of the Cinnabar Moth (*Callimorpha jacobaeae* L.).' The Scientific Management of Animal and Plant Communities for Conservation (Symposium volume), In press.

Dethier, V. G. 1939 'Prothoracic glands of adult Lepidoptera.' *J. NY Entomol. Soc.*, 47: 131.

Ehrlich, P. R. and P. H. Raven 1965 'Butterflies and plants: a study in co-evolution.' *Evolution*, 18: 586.

von Euw, J., L. Fishelson, J. A. Parsons, T. Reichstein and M. Rothschild 1967 'Cardenolides (heart poisons) in a grasshopper feeding on milkweeds.' *Nature (London)*, 214: 35.

Flück, H. 1963 'Intrinsic and extrinsic factors affecting the production of secondary plant products.' *In*: Swain, T. (ed.), *Chemical Plant Taxonomy*, p. 167. Academic Press, New York.

Frazer, J. F. D. and M. Rothschild 1960 'Defence mechanisms in warningly coloured moths and other insects.' *Proc. Eleventh Intern. Congr. Ent. (B)*, 3: 249.

Jones, D. A., J. Parsons and M. Rothschild 1962 'Release of hydrocyanic acid from crushed tissues of all stages in the life-cycle of species of the Zygaeninae (Lepidoptera).' *Nature (London)*, 193: 52.

Klásek, A., T. Reichstein and F. Santavy 1968 'Die Pyrrolizidin-Alkaloide aus *Senecio alpinus* (L.) Scop., *S. subalpinus* Koch und *S. incanus* L. *subsp. carniolicus* (Willd.) Br.-Bl. *Helv. Chim. Acta*, 51: 1088.

Hill, R. K., L. M. Markson and R. Schoental 1960 'Discussion on seneciosis in man and animals.' *Proc. Roy. Soc. Med.*, 53: 281.

Leonard, N. J. 1950; 1960 'Senecio alkaloids.' *In*: Manske, R. H. F. and H. L. Holmes (eds.), *The Alkaloids*. Vol. 1: 107; Vol. 6: 35. Academic Press, New York.

Mattocks, A. R. 1968 'Toxicity of pyrrolizidine alkaloids.' *Nature (London)*, 217: 723.

Neuner-Jehle, N., H. Nesvadba and G. Spiteller 1965 'Anwendung der Massenspektrometrie zur Strukturaufklärung von Alkaloiden, 6 Mitt: Pyrrolizidinalkaloide aus dem Goldregen.' *Monatsh.*, 96: 321.

Reichstein, T., J. von Euw, J. A. Parsons and M. Rothschild 1968 'Heart Poisons in the Monarch Butterfly.' *Science*, 161: 861.

Rothschild, M. 1964 'An extension of Dr Lincoln Brower's theory on bird predation and food specificity, together with some observations on bird memory in relation to aposematic colour patterns.' *Entomologist*, 97: 73.

Rothschild, M. and P. Haskell 1966 'Stridulation of the Garden Tiger Moth (*Arctia caja* L.) audible to the human ear.' *Proc. Roy. Entomol. Soc. London (A)*, 41: 167.

Rothschild, M., T. Reichstein, J. von Euw, R. Aplin and R. R. M. Harman 1971 'Toxic Lepidoptera.' *Toxicon*, **8**: 293.

Schoental, R. and P. N. Magee 1959 'Further observations on the subacute and chronic liver changes in rats after a single dose of various pyrrolizidine (Senecio) alkaloids.' *J. Pathol. Bacteriol.*, **78**: 471.

Self, L. S., F. E. Guthrie and E. Hodgson 1964 'Metabolism of nicotine by tobacco feeding insects.' *Nature (London)*, **204**: 300.

Warren, F. L. 1970 'Senecio Alkaloids.' Manske, R. H. F. (ed.), *In: The Alkaloids*. Vol. **12**: 246. Academic Press, New York.

Wilkinson, A. T. S. 1965 'Release of Cinnabar Moth *Hypocrita jacobaeae* (L.) (Lepidoptera: Arctiidae) on Tansy ragwort in British Columbia.' *Proc. Entomol. Soc. British Columbia*, **62**: 10.

THE CHEMISTRY, PHARMACOLOGY AND TOXICOLOGY OF STEROIDAL GLYCOSIDES

M. E. WALL and K. H. DAVIS, JR

Chemistry and Life Sciences Laboratory, Research Triangle Institute, Research Triangle Park, North Carolina, U.S.A.

INTRODUCTION

THIS PAPER will not attempt to present an exhaustive survey of the various types of saponins and their physiological activity. Instead aspects of the chemistry and biological activity of a selected group of compounds will be discussed. These include the steroidal saponins along with some closely related steroidal alkaloids and some selected examples of triterpenoid saponins.

STEROIDAL SAPONINS AND STEROIDAL ALKALOIDS

Occurrence

The above groups of saponins are found in relatively limited sections of the Plant Kingdom. The occurrence of steroidal saponins is shown in Chart 1, and as indicated, the Order Liliales, comprising the Families Liliaceae, Amaryllidaceae, and Dioscoreaceae, are the main plant groups in which these compounds are found. There are of course exceptions, including the well known saponin digitonin found in *Digitalis lanata*. But, exceptions are relatively few. The distribution of the saponins of steroidal alkaloids is even narrower as all of these compounds are found in the Solanaceae, including

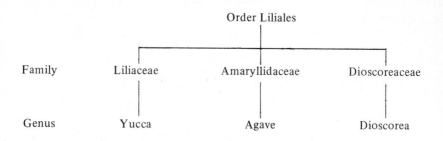

CHART 1   Distribution of steroidal saponins

such common plants as *Solanum tuberosum* (Potato); *S. lycopersicum* (Tomato) and many other related *Solanum* species. Reviews on the steroidal sapogenins and alkaloids can be found in the texts by the Fiesers (1959) and Shoppee (1964). Very detailed studies on the occurrence of steroidal saponins (in the form of their isolated sapogenins) can be found in Marker's classical review of his pioneering studies (1947) and in later reports by Wall and his collaborators (1954a, 1954b, 1955, 1957, 1959). Willaman and Shubert (1961) give a comprehensive review of the occurrence of steroidal alkaloids.

Chemistry

The steroidal saponins consist of a steroid moiety (steroidal sapogenin) linked to a number of sugars. Until recently, methods for purification of the saponins were limited and major attention was paid to the steroidal component, easily obtained by acidic hydrolysis. The classical researches of Marker (1947) established the fact that steroidal sapogenins were C_{27} steroids with a novel spiroketal side chain (Figure 1, X = 0). In particular Marker converted diosgenin to cholesterol, thus showing the interrelationship of the two compounds and constituting the first real demonstration that steroid sapogenins had essentially the same basic carbon skeleton as a well known sterol (Marker and Turner, 1941) (cf. Figure 1). Later work by Wall (1959) and Scheer *et al.* (1955) established the configuration of the spiroketal side chain. As shown in Figure 1, the steroidal sapogenins occur in nature as C_{25} epimers, of which the 25 'iso' or 25D epimer with an equatorial methyl group is the more stable. In addition the surveys by Marker *et al.* (1947) and Wall *et al.* (1954a, 1954b, 1955, 1957, 1959) showed that sapogenins occur with

FIGURE 1   Upper: X = O, Steroidal sapogenin   Lower: Cholesterol
             X = NH, Steroidal alkaloid
             R_1 = H, R_2 = CH_3 = 25D or 25 "iso"
             R_1 = CH_3, R_2 = H = 25L or 25 "neo"

             Fusion of rings A/B may be 5α, 5β or Δ^5.

variations in ring A/B fusion, consisting of 5α, 5β and Δ^5 variants. In addition to a 3β-hydroxyl group, which usually contains the glycosidal linkage, additional hydroxyl groups at positions 1, 2, 5, 6, 12 and 15 have been noted. In addition a 12-keto group is frequently found, particularly in the Agave species (Marker *et al.*, 1947; Wall *et al.*, 1954a, 1954b, 1955, 1957, 1959). Several steroidal sapogenins are of great industrial importance, particularly diosgenin and hecogenin. By a classical process devised by Marker (1940) the spiroketal side chain can readily be degraded to give a 16-dehydropregnene

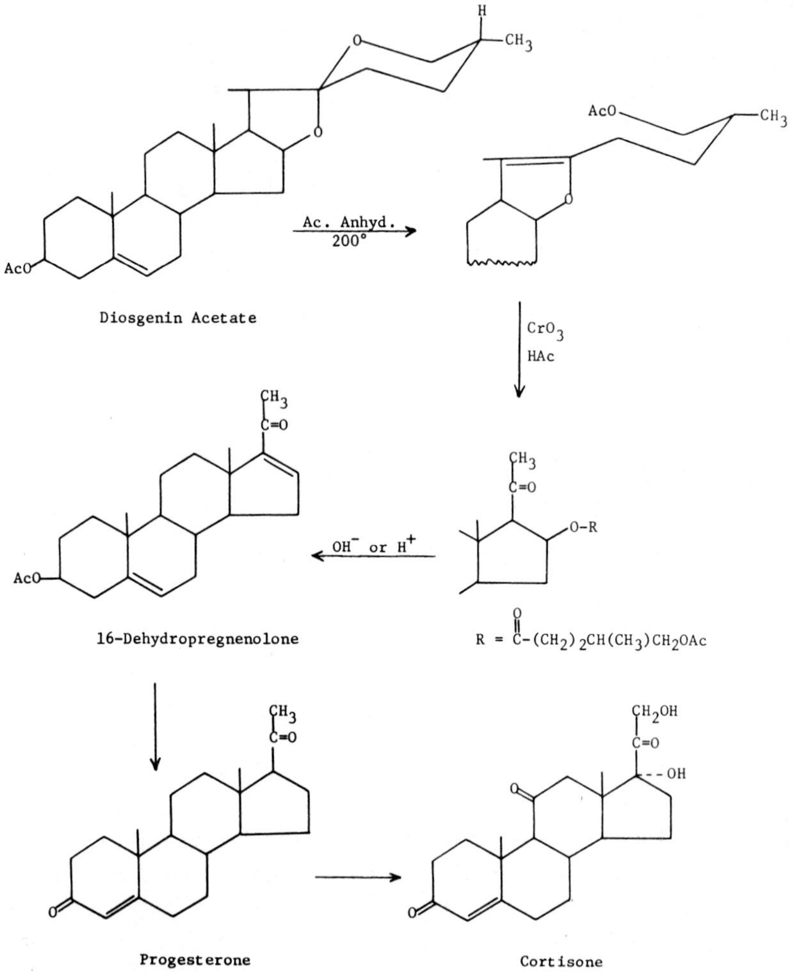

FIGURE 2   Marker's spiroketal sidechain degradation

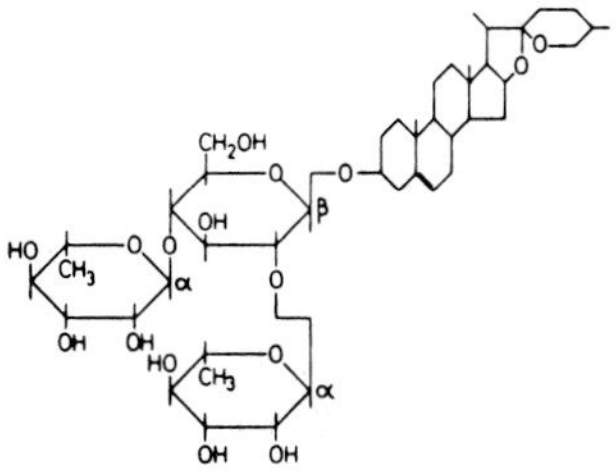

FIGURE 3   Structural formula of steroidal saponin dioscin. (Taken from Birk, 1969)

(cf. Figure 2). By a variety of procedures, including microbiological hydroxylation, these pregnenes can then be converted to all kinds of steroidal hormones (Fieser and Fieser, 1959). In contrast to the steroidal sapogenins, the chemistry of the corresponding saponins is poorly delineated, largely because of the non-crystalline nature of many of the products, their high molecular weight (often > 1000) and until recently, the non-availability of good separation procedures. Krider *et al.* (1955) showed that in the case of sarsasaponin, a crystalline monoglycoside could be obtained by dilute acid hydrolysis thus establishing that at least in this compound the sugars were attached to the 3β-hydroxyl moiety in a linear fashion. The chief sugars found as components in steroidal saponins are glucose, rhamnose, xylose, and arabinose. Kawasaki and Yamauchi (1962) have determined the structure of dioscin (Figure 3). This writer believes that with improved isolation procedures now available (*vide infra*), and with the availability of gas chromatography combined with mass spectrometry for more accurate determination of the individual sugars or their derivatives, that many older saponin analyses (Fieser and Fieser, 1959; Shoppee, 1964) will be revised.

STEROIDAL ALKALOIDS

The chemistry of the steroidal alkaloids is similar to that of the steroidal sapogenins except that nitrogen replaces oxygen in Ring F (cf. Figure 1). L.

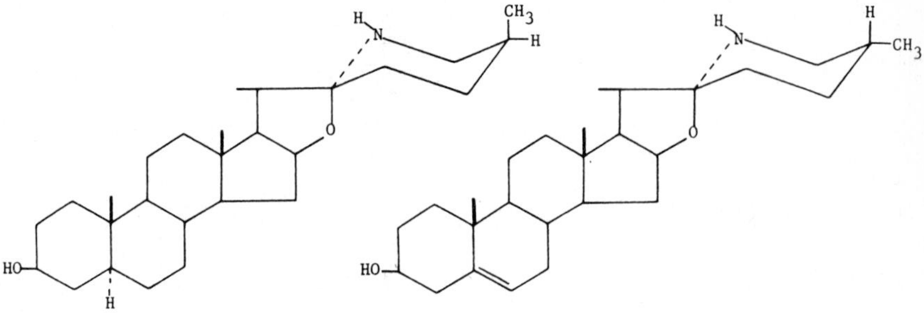

Tomatidine   Solasodine

FIGURE 4   Structures of Tomatidine and Solasodine

H. Briggs and his co-workers in New Zealand were pioneer workers in this field (cf. Fieser and Fieser, 1959, for review). The structures of tomatidine and solasodine, two typical steroidal alkaloids, are shown in Figure 4. These compounds are readily degraded to 16-dehydropregnenes by procedures similar to those used for degradation of the steroidal sapogenin side chain (Sato *et al.*, 1957). The parent saponin of tomatidine is tomatine, isolated in pure form by Fontaine, Irving and co-workers (1948). It is best obtained from wild tomato plants. Tomatine on hydrolysis yields 2 molecules of glucose and one each of galactose and xylose. The antifungal properties of tomatine were of considerable medicinal interest for some years, although currently interest has waned. Solasodine has been of considerable commercial importance, particularly in Eastern Europe because of its facile conversion to $\Delta^{5,16}$-dehydropregnenolone, the basic precursor for many steroidal hormones.

Isolation and analysis of steroidal saponins

There are few general procedures available for this group of compounds. Occasionally, insolubility of certain steroidal saponins in water has permitted their isolation, tomatine for example. A more general procedure has involved a butanol extraction of the glycosides from a previously purified aqueous

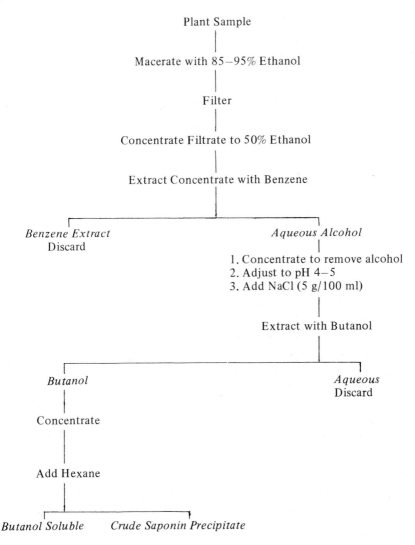

CHART 2   Wall procedure for saponin extraction

solution (Wall *et al.*, 1952b) (cf. Chart 2). More specific procedures can be devised by utilizing anti-tumor assay. Many saponins have an inhibitory effect on the Walker 256-Rat Carcinosarcoma (Kupchan *et al.*, 1967; Wall *et al.*, unpublished data). Charts 3, 4 and 5 show how these assays can be used to

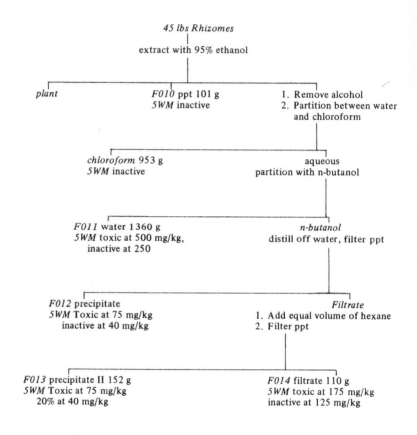

45 lbs Rhizomes
|
extract with 95% ethanol

plant   *F010* ppt 101 g   1. Remove alcohol
                     5WM inactive   2. Partition between water
                                                      and chloroform

          chloroform 953 g   aqueous
          5WM inactive   partition with n-butanol

     F011 water 1 360 g   *n-butanol*
     5WM toxic at 500 mg/kg,   distill off water, filter ppt
     inactive at 250

   F012 precipitate   *Filtrate*
   5WM Toxic at 75 mg/kg   1. Add equal volume of hexane
   inactive at 40 mg/kg   2. Filter ppt

F013 precipitate II 152 g   *F014* filtrate 110 g
5WM Toxic at 75 mg/kg   *5WM* toxic at 175 mg/kg
20% at 40 mg/kg   inactive at 125 mg/kg

Partition chromatography on cellulose using methylethylketone, hexane, methanol and water 70, 10, 10, 10 of 5 grams (F013) yielded 320 mg of *F018* *5WM* 34% at 15 mg/kg

Sephadex LH−20 chromatography on 150 mg of *F018* yielded

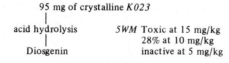

        95 mg of crystalline *K023*
        |
acid hydrolysis   *5WM* Toxic at 15 mg/kg
        | 28% at 10 mg/kg
   Diosgenin   inactive at 5 mg/kg

CHART 3   Isolation of steroidal saponin from *Trillium erectum*   B620802

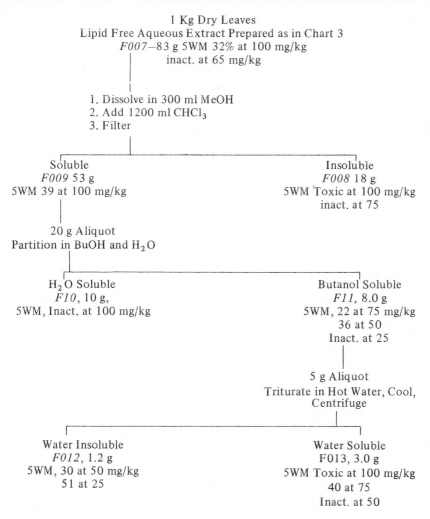

1 Kg Dry Leaves
Lipid Free Aqueous Extract Prepared as in Chart 3
F007–83 g 5WM 32% at 100 mg/kg
inact. at 65 mg/kg

1. Dissolve in 300 ml MeOH
2. Add 1200 ml $CHCl_3$
3. Filter

Soluble
F009 53 g
5WM 39 at 100 mg/kg

Insoluble
F008 18 g
5WM Toxic at 100 mg/kg
inact. at 75

20 g Aliquot
Partition in BuOH and H_2O

H_2O Soluble
F10, 10 g,
5WM, Inact. at 100 mg/kg

Butanol Soluble
F11, 8.0 g
5WM, 22 at 75 mg/kg
36 at 50
Inact. at 25

5 g Aliquot
Triturate in Hot Water, Cool,
Centrifuge

Water Insoluble
F012, 1.2 g
5WM, 30 at 50 mg/kg
51 at 25

Water Soluble
F013, 3.0 g
5WM Toxic at 100 mg/kg
40 at 75
Inact. at 50

CHART 4   Isolation of steroidal saponin from *Agave brandeegii* Trel,
B604578

isolate saponins, which appear to be pure as judged by thin layer chromatography. Analyses for saponins have been devised which take advantage of their hemolytic or foaming properties. The procedures at best are inexact and non-specific. An excellent review by Birk is found in a recent treatise on chemistry and toxicology of saponins (Birk, 1969). Usually a saponin can

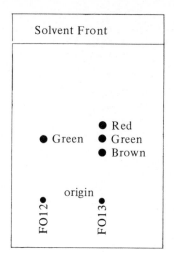

CHART 5   Thin layer chromatography and analysis of *Agave brandeegi* saponins

TLC System BuOH, HAC, H_2O, Ratio 5:1:4
The upper phase of this system is used for TLC development.
Spots were detected with a ceric sulfate/sulfuric acid spray.

HCl hydrolysis of F012 gives tigogenin

Sugar analysis of alditol acetates by Glc

1—Rhamnose

4—Xylose   Calculated M.W. of saponin
                          2,370
2—Galactose

6—Glucose

best be analyzed in terms of its constituents obtained by acid hydrolysis. Thus Wall *et al.* (1952a) have devised infrared procedures for the analysis of crude steroidal sapogenins. The sugars can best be estimated on hydrolyzates of reasonably well purified saponins by thin layer or gas chromatography. Figure 5 presents a gas-liquid chromatogram of the sugars obtained from the pure saponin of *Agave brandeegii*. The sugars were converted to the

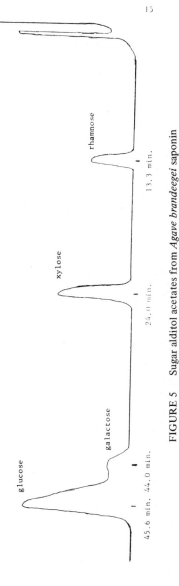

FIGURE 5   Sugar alditol acetates from *Agave brandeegei* saponin

6′ – 3% FCNSS-M
Injector – 210°
Detector – 200°
Column – 140° programmed at 0.5°/min.

corresponding alditol acetates by sodium borohydride reduction, followed by acetylation using the procedure of Crowell and Burnett (1967) as modified in our laboratory (Abernethy and Wall, unpublished data).

TRITERPENOID SAPONINS

Occurrence

In contrast to the relatively narrow distribution of steroidal saponins, the triterpenoid saponins are virtually ubiquitous being found in a wide variety of dicotyledonous plants. Interestingly, they do not occur in the monocotyledonous Liliales Order which contain the steroidal saponins. Many common economic plants which are used as human or animal feedstuffs contain triterpenoid saponins (Birk, 1969) including such common plants as alfalfa, soybean, spinach, beets, sugar beets, clovers, yams, and tea. In this report because of obvious space and time limitations, we will discuss only our work on alfalfa saponins (Davis and Wall, 1970). The general field with particular emphasis on alfalfa and soybean saponins has been very well reviewed by Birk (1969). The saponin content of alfalfa varies with the plant part and the variety. Table 1 (Davis and Wall, 1970) compares the DuPuits (high saponin) and Lahontan (low saponin) varieties by the carbon adsorption procedure devised by Van Atta *et al.* (1961). The greatest differences were in the leaves of DuPuits variety which consistently showed almost twice the saponin content of Lahontan variety. Flowers and roots which contained in the neighbourhood of 2.5–3.5% saponin contained the highest amounts, stems were lowest with about 0.5% content. The seeds did not contain high amounts, about 1.2–1.5%. This is in contrast to Wall's findings with *Yucca* and *Agave* seeds which contained huge quantities of saponin, 10–20 fold higher than other plant parts.

Chemistry

The aglycones of the triterpenoid saponins contain 30 carbon atoms and are pentacyclic compounds derived from oleanan. The common tetracyclic triterpenoids are usually found in the free aglycone form in nature and will not be discussed in this paper. A comprehensive review of the triterpenoid saponins is given by Boiteau *et al.* (1964). The carbohydrates are usually but not always, linked to the triterpenoid skeleton by glycosidic linkages at C_2 or C_3.

TABLE 1   Data from the carbon adsorption analysis of alfalfa collections

Variety	Plant Part	USDA Log No.	% Saponin
DuPuits	flowers	143	3.73
Lahontan	flowers	144	2.95
DuPuits	leaves	139	1.88
Lahontan	leaves	141	1.15
DuPuits	leaves	183	1.91
Lahontan	leaves	185	1.15
DuPuits	leaves	196	2.04
Lahontan	leaves	199	1.11
DuPuits	stems	140	0.56
Lahontan	stems	142	0.43
DuPuits	stems	182	0.62
DuPuits	stems	197	0.58
Lahontan	stems	200	0.43
DuPuits	seeds	–	1.22
Lahontan	seeds	–	1.50
DuPuits	pods	194	1.90
Lahontan	pods	193	1.61
DuPuits	roots	198	2.56
Lahontan	roots	201	3.43
DuPuits	whole plant	137	1.79
DuPuits	whole plant	202	1.55
Lahontan	whole plant	203	1.01
Lahontan	whole plant	209	1.39
DuPuits	whole plant	210	1.43

Structure of alfalfa saponins

As with their steroidal counterparts, the structure of alfalfa saponins is known in terms of its constituents found on hydrolysis. A number of triterpenoid pentacyclic sapogenins of known structure have been isolated from acid hydrolyzed alfalfa saponins including soyasapogenol A,B,C,D and medicagenic acid (Figure 6) (cf. Birk, 1969, for literature review). In addition Livingston (1959) has isolated lucernic acid, a compound of only partially known structure. The usual hexoses, pentoses, uronic acids have been noted

Oleanan

in the sugars (Birk, 1969). No data is as yet available on the full saponin structure or order of linkage of the sugars.

Isolation of alfalfa saponins

Our general procedure for the isolation of crude alfalfa saponins is based on a final butanol-water partition (Chart 6). As was the case for the steroidal saponins, the butanol removes most of the saponin from water. Subsequently various saponin precipitates can be obtained by partial concentration and cooling of the butanol solution. Most of the saponins obtained in this manner are mixtures of at least 6 or more components. Figure 7 shows an analytical thin layer chromatogram which compares the butanol precipitates of standard DuPuits and Lahontan leaf meal saponin extracts. Referring to Figure 7, the numbers I–IV represent crude saponins of *increasing* butanol solubility. Six components, called AA–E are routinely found, and a seventh, between D and E is frequently noted. It will be noted that components C,D are absent or very small in the more soluble fractions. In general there was little qualitative difference between the DuPuits and Lahontan precipitates. Of interest, also, was the fact that a saponin prepared by cholesterol precipitation (Walter *et al.*, 1954) does not contain components AA or E. Birk (1969, p. 179) reports unpublished studies which show that alfalfa saponins purified in a somewhat different manner had as many as 8 components. Figure 8 shows a similar study, based on one major butanol precipitate, of the various alfalfa plant parts. In general flowers, leaves, stems and roots show similarity. Noteably different are the seeds.

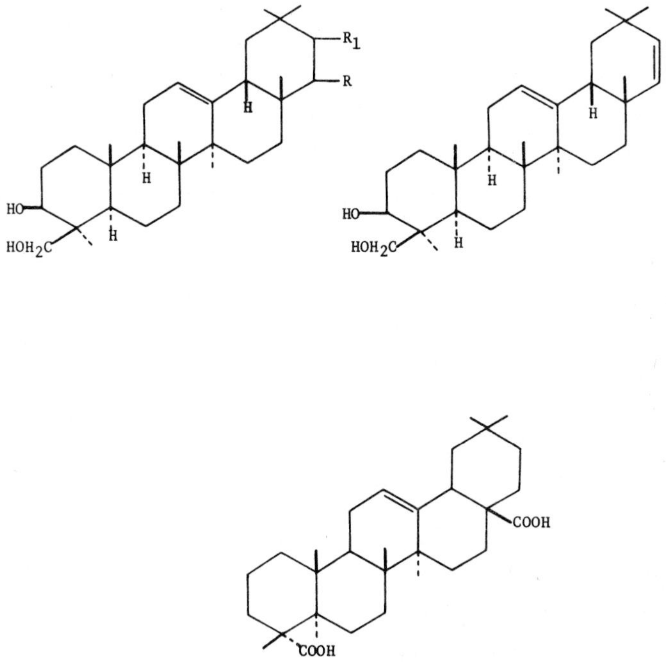

FIGURE 6   Structure of alfalfa sapogenins

Upper: Soyasapogenol A, R = R$_1$ = —OH   Lower: Medicagenic acid
Soyasapogenol B, R = H, R$_1$ = —OH
Soyasapogenol E, R = H, R$_1$ = -O

Further purification of alfalfa saponins

We have undertaken additional studies to see if the complex saponin mixture can be further purified by column chromatography so that appreciable, i.e. 50–100 mg quantities of highly purified saponins could be obtained. Using silica gel (Davison Chemical Co., Baltimore, Md.,) 100–200 mesh, in a 1000/1 ratio to the weight of the saponin mixture and acetonitrile, acetic acid, water mixture as an eluant, ratios of 85:5:10 initially, with slowly increasing water and acetic acid gradients, partial separation of the saponin

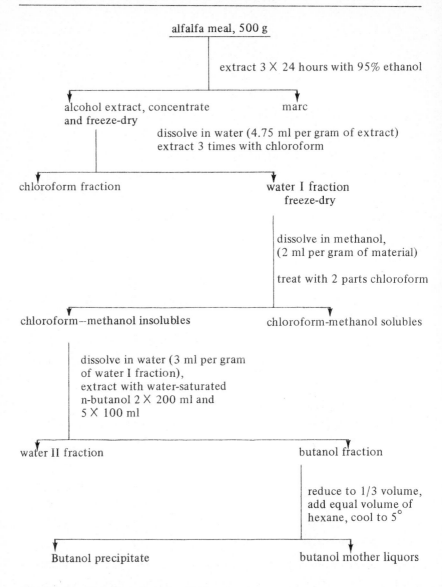

CHART 6   Isolation of crude alfalfa saponin

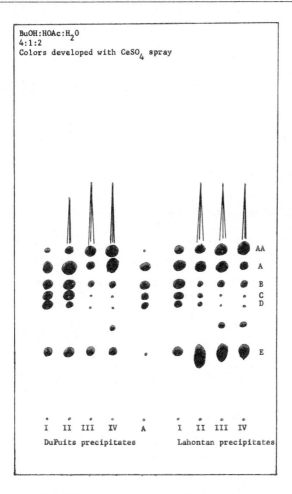

FIGURE 7   Analytical thin-layer chromatogram of various butanol precipitates from DuPuits and Lahontan saponins

A = DuPuits cholesteride saponin

components could be achieved. Figure 9 shows the analytical TLC data found for a typical silica gel separation. It can be seen that the six-component mixture has been resolved into a number of fractions, usually binary mixtures, of increasing polarity. It should be stated that the highly polar and acidic eluant used extracts a number of low molecular weight impurities

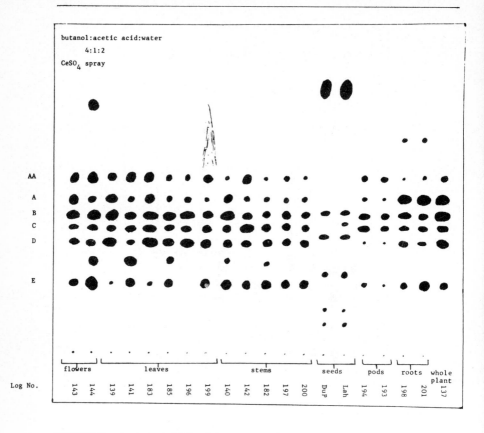

FIGURE 8   Analytical TLC of butanol precipitates from DuPuits and Lahontan plant fractions

from the silica gel. Passing these binary mixtures through a column of Sephadex G-15 completely removes silica gel impurities and has further resolved some of the saponin mixtures. Saponins B, E and D have been obtained in pure form with the following optical rotations ($[\alpha]_D^{25}$, H_2O) respectively: $-11.4°$, $+28.6°$, and $-1.4°$. Obviously B and E must differ greatly.

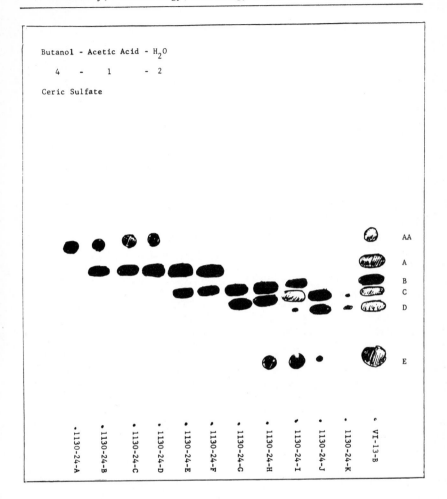

FIGURE 9   Analytical TLC of silica gel chromatography fractions obtained from Lahontan butanol precipitate

IDENTIFICATION OF AGLUCONES AND INDIVIDUAL SUGARS FROM SAPONIN HYDROLYZATES

Aglucones

Butanol precipitate fractions representing saponins obtained from extraction

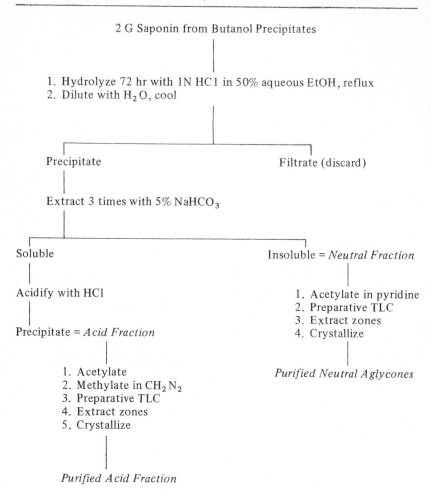

2 G Saponin from Butanol Precipitates

1. Hydrolyze 72 hr with 1N HC1 in 50% aqueous EtOH, reflux
2. Dilute with H_2O, cool

Precipitate   Filtrate (discard)

Extract 3 times with 5% $NaHCO_3$

Soluble   Insoluble = *Neutral Fraction*

Acidify with HCl   1. Acetylate in pyridine
                                           2. Preparative TLC
                                           3. Extract zones
Precipitate = *Acid Fraction*   4. Crystallize

1. Acetylate   *Purified Neutral Aglycones*
2. Methylate in CH_2N_2
3. Preparative TLC
4. Extract zones
5. Crystallize

Purified Acid Fraction

CHART 7   Isolation and analysis of aglycones from alfalfa saponin

of a sample of DuPuits whole plant alfalfa meal were hydrolyzed in 1N ethanolic HCl by the method of Djerassi *et al.* (1957). Chart 7 gives an outline of the procedure. We have found it preferable to divide the aglycones into neutral and acidic fractions. The neutral and acidic compounds are then acetylated, the latter being also converted to methyl esters. Table 2 shows the

TABLE 2   High resolution mass spectrometry data on alfalfa aglycones

Compound	Molecular Formula	m/e, Calculated	m/e, Found
Soyasapogenol A tetra-acetate	$C_{38}H_{58}O_8$	642.4131	642.4176
Soyasapogenol B triacetate	$C_{36}H_{56}O_6$	584.4077	584.4059
Unknown acetate	$C_{23}H_{20}O_{10}$	456.1056	456.1065
Diacetoxy dimethyl medicagenate	$C_{36}H_{54}O_8$	614.3819	614.3856
Triacetoxy methyl lucernate	$C_{37}H_{54}O_{10}$	658.3717	658.3771

five compounds isolated to date, their molecular formulae and high resolution mass spectrometry data obtained. One of the compounds, the 'unknown acetate,' is obviously not a triterpenoid. Other aglycones not shown in Table 2 are also present, but in small quantity, and have not been fully purified to date.

Sugars

In order to obtain good results on sugars in saponin hydrolysis, another method of hydrolysis was used. In this procedure based on the method of Saeman et al. (1954), a 32 milligram sample of saponin is dissolved in 0.3 milliliters of 72% sulfuric acid. After standing 1 hour, more water is added (9 X dilution) and the solution is heated on a steam bath for 1 hour. After cooling and neutralizing, the rest of the procedure is identical to an alditol acetate method, described under Steroidal Saponins. Rhamnose, arabinose, xylose and glucose have been identified. Figure 10 gives a typical gas-liquid chromatograph obtained on a highly purified alfalfa saponin.

Pharmacology and toxicology of saponins

This section will deal with both the steroidal and triterpenoid saponins as the biological properties of these compounds are closely related. All saponins, whether steroidal or triterpenoid, hemolyze red blood cells, probably because

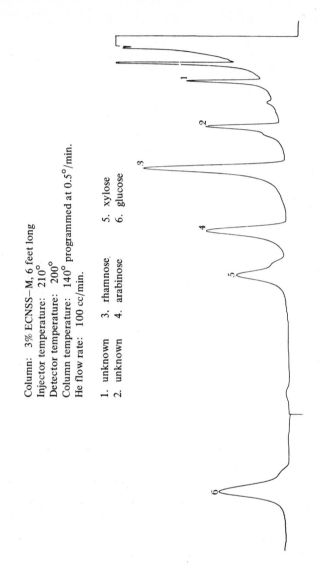

Column: 3% ECNSS—M, 6 feet long
Injector temperature: 210°
Detector temperature: 200°
Column temperature: 140° programmed at 0.5°/min.
He flow rate: 100 cc/min.

1. unknown   3. rhamnose   5. xylose
2. unknown   4. arabinose   6. glucose

FIGURE 10   GLC of saponin B sugar alditol acetates

of their surface active nature (Fieser and Fieser, 1959; Shoppee, 1964; Birk, 1969). They are extremely toxic to cold blooded animals and have been for centuries used as fish poisons.

Alfalfa saponins (triterpenoid) have been extensively studied since alfalfa leaf meal is extensively used in chicken and animal feedstuffs. Alfalfa saponin

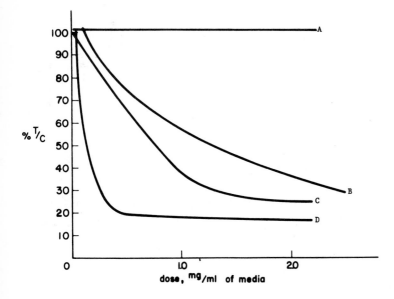

FIGURE 11   The effect of crude Lahontan and DuPuits saponin preparations on the growth of *Trichoderma viride* Pers. ex Fr.

A - Lahontan water extract (meal previously extracted with 95% alcohol)
B - DuPuits water extract (meal previously extracted with 95% alcohol)
C - Lahontan butanol precipitate I
D - DuPuits butanol precipitate I

inhibits the germination of cotton seed (Pedersen, 1965) and lettuce seed (Pedersen *et al.*, 1967), and also inhibits the growth of the fungus *Trichoderma viride* (Pedersen *et al.*, 1966). The latter property can be utilized as a convenient assay during the purification of alfalfa saponin. Figure 11 shows some data obtained in our laboratory using a slight modification of Pederson's procedures (Pedersen *et al.,* 1966, 1967). It will be noted from Figure 11 that saponin obtained from the DuPuits variety is much more inhibitory to the growth of *T. viride* than are comparable Lahontan fractions. At present insufficient data is available to determine whether this difference in inhibition is due to the quantitative difference in saponin content (it will be recalled that in general the DuPuits variety is higher in total saponin than

Lahontan) or to a particular constituent. In Figure 11, fractions C and D are both purified saponins (although a multi-component mixture). Yet on an equal weight basis DuPuits is much more inhibitory.

The effects of alfalfa meal and alfalfa saponins on the growth of chicks and egg production have been intensively studied because of the widespread use of alfalfa meal in commercial chick diets. Although saponins added to the diet in 0.2–0.4% by various investigators (cf. Birk, 1969, for literature review) do indeed inhibit chick growth and depress egg laying, there seems to be little effect at the level of alfalfa meal normally used in chick feed rations, i.e. 3–5%, which would be equivalent to 0.1% alfalfa saponin at a maximum. Wilson and co-workers (1957) found that in the case of the rat, toxicity by oral administration was much less than by the intravenous route. Birk (1969) in her comprehensive review quoting her studies and those of Gestetner on alfalfa and soybean saponins, conclude that oral administration of these saponins is essentially harmless, largely because they are not absorbed from the intestines. Oser (1966) found that the saponin from *Yucca mohavensis* (steroidal saponin), which is used as a foaming agent in rootbeer, had no effect on growth and various clinical analyses conducted on young albino rats.

During the course of isolating a number of pure saponins with antitumor activity, we were able, probably for the first time, to obtain some lethality data with highly purified saponins of every type. The data is shown in Chart 8. In every case the animal used was the rat and the route of administration intraperitoneal. The data shown in Chart 8 is that many of these saponins are quite lethal when administered in this manner. The writers cannot accept the theory that saponins in general are innocuous compounds. In particular the use of these in beverages should be closely controlled or hopefully replaced.

ACKNOWLEDGMENTS

Studies reported in this paper which deal with antitumor activity from plant saponins have been supported under contract No. NIH 69–2019, Cancer Chemotherapy National Service Center, National Cancer Institute, National Institutes of Health. The work on alfalfa saponins was supported under contract No. 12–14–100–8930(34), U.S. Department of Agriculture.

Plant	Dose (mg/kg)	Survivors	T/C*
Agave brandegeeii			
Purified saponin, F012	100	0/4	
Steroid sap. → tigogenin	75	2/4	
	50	4/4	30
	25	4/4	51
Hesperaloe parviflora			
Purified saponin, K028	25	0/4	
Steroid sap. → tigogenin	15	0/4	
	10	2/4	
	5	4/4	27
Trillium erectum			
Purified saponin, K023	15	1/4	
Steroid sap. → Diosgenin	10	4/4	28
	5	4/4	67
	3	4/4	86
Solanum marginatum			
Purified saponin, F050	50		30
Steroid. alk. → solasodine	25		53
Ipomopsis aggregata			
Purified saponin, F108	20	0/4	
Triterpenoid saponin	10	0/4	
	5	4/4	35
	3	4/4	64
Acer pennsylvanicum			
Purified saponin, F068	50	0/4	
Structure unknown,	25	0/4	
probably triterpenoid	15	4/4	38
	10	4/4	69

CHART 8   Effect of saponins on rat mortality and tumor inhibition of Walker 256 Carcinosarcoma

*An active tumor inhibition is regarded as a Test/Control Ratio of 0.42 or less. Parameter measured is tumor weight.

SUMMARY

The compounds discussed in this paper include the glycosides of steroidal sapogenins, steroidal alkaloids, and steroidal triterpenes. The cardiac glycosides will not be discussed. The general chemical features of each of the classes are described. General methods for the isolation of these compounds are discussed, along with a brief description of newer analytical procedures, in particular thin layer chromatography, gas-liquid chromatography and mass spectrometry.

The pharmacology and toxicology of the various groups of compounds are discussed. Such properties as hemolytic activity, fish poisons, effects of alfalfa saponins on the chick and LD_{50} data are discussed in some detail. In particular the antitumor activity of some of these compounds are described.

References

Birk, Y. 1969 Saponins, in: *'Toxic Constituents of Plant Foodstuffs.'* Liener, I. E. (ed.), pp. 169—210. Academic Press, New York.

Boiteau, P., B. Pasich and A. Rakoto Ratsimamanga 1964 'Les Triterpénoides en Physiologie Végétale et Animale.' Gauthier-Villars, (ed.), Centre National de la Recherche Scientifique, Paris.

Crowell, E. P. and B. B. Burnett 1967 'Determination of the carbohydrate composition of wood pulps by gas chromatography of the alditol acetates.' *Anal. Chem.,* **39**: 121—124.

Davis, K. H., Jr and M. E. Wall 1970 Final Report. 'Investigations on the relationship of saponins to pest resistance in alfalfa.' USDA Contract No. 12—14—100—8930(34) (May 1967—May 1969).

Djerassi, C., D. B. Thomas, A. L. Livingston and C. R. Thompson 1957 'Terpenoids. XXXI. The structure and stereochemistry of medicagenic acid.' *J. Amer. Chem. Soc.,* **79**: 5292—5297.

Fieser, L. F. and M. Fieser 1959 *'Steroids.'* Reinhold Publishing Corp., New York. pp. 810—895.

Fontaine, T. D., G. W. Irving, Jr, R. Ma, J. B. Poole and S. P. Doolittle 1948 'Isolation and partial characterization of crystalline tomatine, an antibiotic agent from the tomato plant.' *Arch. Biochem.,* **18**: 467—475.

Kawasaki, T. and T. Yamauchi 1962 'Structures of dioscin, gracillin, and kikuba-saponin (Saponins of Japanese Dioscoreaceae). XI.' *Chem. Pharm. Bull.,* **10**: 703—708.

Krider, M. M., J. R. Branaman and M. E. Wall 1955 'Steroidal Sapogenins. XVIII. Partial hydrolysis of steroidal saponins of *Yucca Schidigera.*' *J. Amer. Chem. Soc.,* **77**: 1238—1241.

Kupchan, S. M., R. J. Hemingway, J. R. Knox, S. J. Barboutis, D. Werner and M. A. Barboutis 1967 'Tumor inhibitors. XXI. Active principles of *Acer negundo* and *Cyclamen persicum.'* *J. Pharm. Sci.,* **56**: 603—608.

Livingston, A. L. 1959 'Lucernic acid, a new triterpene from alfalfa.' *J. Org. Chem.,* **24**: 1567—1568.

Marker, R. E. 1940 'Sterols. CXIII. Sapogenins. XLII. The conversion of the sapogenins to the pregnenolones.' *J. Amer. Chem. Soc.,* **62**: 3350—3352.

Marker, R. E. and D. L. Turner 1941 'The relation between diosgenin and cholesterol.' *J. Amer. Chem. Soc.,* **63**: 767—771.

Marker, R. E., R. B. Wagner, P. R. Ulshafer, E. L. Wittbecker, D. P. J. Goldsmith and C. H. Ruof 1947 'Steroidal sapogenins.' *J. Amer. Chem. Soc.,* **69**: 2167—2230.

Oser, B. L. 1966 'An evaluation of *Yucca mohavensis* as a source of food grade saponin.' *Food Cosmet. Toxicol.,* **4**: 57—61.

Pedersen, M. W. 1965 'Effect of alfalfa saponin on cottonseed germination.' *J. Agron.,* **57**: 516—517.

Pedersen, M. W., D. E. Zimmer, D. R. McAllister, J. O. Anderson, M. D. Wilding, G. A. Taylor and C. F. McGuire 1967 'Comparative studies of saponin of several alfalfa varieties using chemical and biochemical assays.' *Crop Sci.,* **7**: 349—352.

Pedersen, M. W., D. E. Zimmer, J. O. Anderson and C. F. McGuire 1966 'A comparison of saponins from DuPuits, Lahontan, Ranger and Uinta alfalfas.' Proc. X Intern. Grassland Cong. Helsinki, pp. 693—698.

Saeman, J. F., W. E. Moore, R. L. Mitchell and M. A. Millett 1954 'Techniques for the determination of pulp constituents by qualitative paper chromatography.' *Tappi*, **37**: 336–343.

Sato, Y. H. G. Latham, Jr and E. Mosettig 1957 'Some reactions of solasodine.' *J. Org. Chem.*, **22**: 1496–1500.

Scheer, I., R. B. Kostic and E. Mosettig 1955 'The C-25 isomerization of smilagenin and sarsasapogenin.' *J. Amer. Chem. Soc.*, **77**: 641–646.

Shoppee, C. W. 1964 *'Chemistry of the Steroids.'* 2nd Ed. Butterworths, London. pp. 398–432.

Van Atta, G. R., J. Guggolz and C. R. Thompson 1961 'Determination of saponins in alfalfa.' *J. Agr. Food. Chem.*, **9**: 77–79.

Wall, M. E. 1959 'Steroidal sapogenins. XXX. Stereochemistry of the side chain.' *Experientia*, **11**: 340–341.

Wall, M. E., C. R. Eddy, M. L. McClennan and M. E. Klumpp 1952a 'Steroidal sapogenins. II. Detection and estimation of steroidal sapogenins in plant tissue.' *Anal. Chem.*, **24**: 1337–1341.

Wall, M. E., C. R. Eddy, J. J. Willaman, D. S. Correll, B. G. Schubert and H. S. Gentry 1954b 'Steroidal sapogenins. XII. Survey of plants for steroidal sapogenins and other constituents.' *J. Amer. Pharm. Assoc. (Sci. Ed.)*, **43**: 503–505.

Wall, M. E., C. S. Fenske, J. W. Garvin, J. J. Willaman, Q. Jones, B. G. Schubert and H. S. Gentry 1959 'Steroidal sapogenins. LV. Survey of plants for steroidal sapogenins and other constituents. *J. Amer. Pharm. Assoc. (Sci. Ed.)*, **48**: 695–722.

Wall, M. E., C. S. Fenske, H. E. Kenney, J. J. Willaman, D. S. Correll, B. G. Schubert and H. S. Gentry 1957 'Steroidal sapogenins. XLIII. Survey of plants for steroidal sapogenins and other constituents.' *J. Amer. Pharm. Assoc. (Sci. Ed.)*, **46**: 653–686.

Wall, M. E., C. S. Fenske, J. J. Willaman, D. S. Correll, B. G. Schubert and H. S. Gentry 1955 'Steroidal sapogenins. XXV. Survey of plants for steroidal sapogenins and other constituents.' *J. Amer. Pharm. Assoc. (Sci. Ed.)*, **44**: 438–440.

Wall, M. E., M. M. Krider, C. F. Krewson, C. R. Eddy, J. J. Willaman, D. S. Correll and H. S. Gentry 1954a 'Steroidal sapogenins. VII. Survey of plants for steroidal sapogenins and other constituents.' *J. Amer. Pharm. Assoc. (Sci. Ed.)*, **43**: 1–7.

Wall, M. E., M. M. Krider, E. S. Rothman and C. R. Eddy 1952b 'Steroidal sapogenins. I. Extraction, isolation and identification.' *J. Biol. Chem.*, **198**: 533–543.

Walter, E. D., G. R. Van Atta, C. R. Thompson and W. D. Maclay 1954 'Alfalfa saponin.' *J. Amer. Chem. Soc.*, **76**: 2271–2273.

Willaman, J. J. and B. G. Schubert 1961 'Alkaloid-bearing plants and their contained alkaloids.' *U.S. Dept. Agr. Tech. Bull.* No. **1234**, Washington, D. C.

Wilson, R. H., M. B. Sidemann and F. De Eds 1957 In: 'Some pharmacological effects of alfalfa saponin on nonruminants and on isolated muscle strips. Alfalfa saponins. Studies on their chemical, pharmacological and physiological properties in relation to ruminant bloat.' pp. 70–81. *U.S. Dept. Agr. Tech. Bull.* No. **1161**, Washingotn, D. C.

AMINO ACID SEQUENCES AND DISULFIDE BONDS OF SMALL TOXIC PROTEINS FROM PLANTS OF THE FAMILY LORANTHACEAE

G. SAMUELSSON, TH. OLSON, T. MELLSTRAND
and B. PETTERSSON

*Department of Pharmacognosy, Faculty of Pharmacy,
Stockholm, Sweden*

THE EUROPEAN MISTLETOE, *Viscum album*, contains several small, basic proteins with a molecular weight of about 5,000. These substances were first isolated as a mixture by Winterfeld and Bijl (1948) and given the name Viscotoxin. We have developed an isolation method for the Viscotoxins comprising the following steps: An aqueous extract of the dried plant material is passed through a column of the cation exchanger IRC 50 H^+ which adsorbs the basic proteins. Following elution with 0.1 N HCl and exchange of HCl for HOAc by the anion exchanger IR 45 the proteins are precipitated with cold acetone and separated from salts and other small molecules by gel-filtration on Sephadex G-25 (Samuelsson, 1961). The protein fraction is chromatographed on phosphate cellulose (Samuelsson, 1966) and sulphoethyl Sephadex (Samuelsson and Pettersson, 1970) yielding three pure proteins: Viscotoxin A2, Viscotoxin A3 and Viscotoxin B. Parenterally administrated these proteins produce reflex bradycardia, negative inotropic effects on the heart muscle, hypotension and, in high doses, vasoconstriction of vessels in the skin and skeletal muscle. The intravenous lethal dose of Viscotoxin A3 is about 0.1 mg/kg of bodyweight in cats (Rosell and Samuelsson, 1966). Using conventional methods involving breaking of the disulfide bonds by performic acid oxidation, enzymatic degradation and

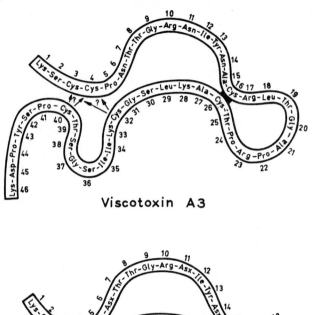

Viscotoxin A3

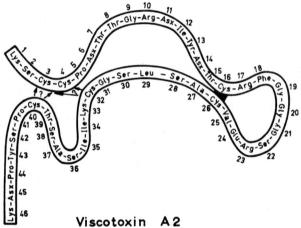

Viscotoxin A2

FIGURE 1.   Amino acid sequence of Viscotoxin

Edman degradation of separated peptides, the amino acid sequence of Visco-toxin A3 (Samuelsson *et al.*, 1968) and Viscotoxin A2 have been determined (Figure 1). The determination of the amino acid sequence of Viscotoxin B is in progress and the results indicate that this protein is very much like Visco-toxin A2, the differences being that amino acid No. 18 is Leu instead of Phe and No 25 is Arg instead of Val.

As seen in Figure 1 the disulfide bonds of Viscotoxin A2 and A3 are the same. We have not yet been able to decide whether each of the residues Cys 3 or Cys 4 is linked to Cys 32 or to Cys 40. In order to solve this problem the peptide linkage between Cys 3 and Cys 4 must be broken leaving the SS bridges intact. The only method available for this is partial acid hydrolysis which, however, yields a large number of fragments. Partly due to lack of sufficient amounts of material we have not yet been able to isolate a key fragment from the peptide mixture formed by partial acid hydrolysis.

Screening of 41 different species of mistletoes for Viscotoxin-like proteins has revealed the presence of such substances in 5 species, all within the sub-family Viscoideae. From one of these plants, *Phoradendron tomentosum* (DC) Engelman subsp. *macrophyllum* (Cockerell) Wiens (= *Phoradendron serotinum* (Raf.) M.C. Johnst.)—a pure protein has been isolated and given the name Phoratoxin (Samuelsson and Ekblad, 1967). Phoratoxin has the same pharmacological effects as the Viscotoxins. Also this substance is composed of 46 amino acids and the chain is bridged by 3 disulfide bonds. Tryptic digestion of the performic acid oxidized material yielded 8 fragments the amino acid sequences of which are:

T1: Lys

T2: Ser-Cys(SO_3H)-Cys(SO_3H)-Pro-Thr-Thr-Thr-Ala-Arg

T3: Asx-Ile-Tyr-Asx-Thr-Cys(SO_3)H-Arg

T4: Phe-Gly-Gly-Gly-Ser-Arg

T5: Pro-Val-Cys(SO_3H)-Ala-Lys

T6: Leu-Ser-Gly-Cys(SO_3H)-Lys

T7: Ile-Ile-Ser-Gly-Thr-Lys

T8: Cys(SO_3H)-Asx-Ser-(modified Trp, Asx, Gly, His)

  (Asx=Asp or Asn).

The sequence of the first 4 amino acids in the N-terminal part of Phoratoxin is Lys-Ser-Cys-Cys. There are many similarities between these sequences and those of the Viscotoxins. Thus the sequence of the first 6 amino acids of fragment T2 is the same as the sequence of amino acids 2—8 in the Viscotoxins. Fragment T3 and T4 corresponds to the sequence 11—23 of Viscotoxin A2. Fragment T6 and the first 4 amino acids of fragment T7 correspond to the sequence of amino acids 29—37 of Viscotoxin A3.

The facts so far known about the structure of this group of small proteins are too few to permit a serious attempt at deduction of a structure-pharmacological effect relationship, but some speculations might be permissible. Thus it is evident that the disulfide bridges are necessary for the preservation of the toxic effects as the oxidized material is completely inactive. The presence of two peptide linked Cys residues in the N-terminal part of the chain is a common feature for all the substances studied and might be important in securing a rigid secondary structure through the disulfide bridges to Cys residues in the C-terminal part of the chain. It is also noteworthy that all arginine residues are present in the N-terminal part of the chains and that all Lys residues are confined to the C-terminal part.

ACKNOWLEDGMENTS

This work has been supported by grants from the Swedish Medical Science Research Council (Projects No. B 68—13x—2084—02, B 69—13x—2084—03A, B 70—13x—2084—04B).

SUMMARY

The European mistletoe, *Viscum album* L., contains several small, basic proteins with a molecular weight around 5000. These substances were first isolated as a mixture, which was given the name Viscotoxin. By chromatography on cellulose phosphate and sulfoethyl Sephadex[R] the pure substances Viscotoxin A2, Viscotoxin A3 and Viscotoxin B have been isolated. Parenterally administered, these proteins produce reflex bradycardia, negative inotropic effect on the heart, hypotension and, in high doses, vasoconstriction of vessels in the skin and skeletal muscle. The intravenous lethal dose of viscotoxin is about 0.1 mg/kg of body weight (cat). The amino acid sequences of Viscotoxin A2 and Viscotoxin A3 are shown below. Both substances contain 46 amino acids and the sequences are identical for amino acids 1—14, 16, 17, 20, 23, 26, 27, 29—36, and 38—46.

```
Viscotoxin A2:  Lys-Ser-Cys-Cys-Pro-Asx-Thr-Thr-Gly-Arg-
Viscotoxin A3:  Lys-Ser-Cys-Cys-Pro-Asn-Thr-Thr-Gly-Arg-
                 1    2    3    4    5    6    7    8    9   10

Asx-Ile-Tyr-Asx-Thr-Cys-Arg-Phe-Gly-Gly-Gly-Ser-Arg-Glu-
Asn-Ile-Tyr-Asn-Ala-Cys-Arg-Leu-Thr-Gly-Ala-Pro-Arg-Pro-
 11   12   13   14   15   16   17   18   19   20   21   22   23   24

Val-Cys-Ala-Ser-Leu-Ser-Gly-Cys-Lys-Ile-Ile-Ser-Ala-Ser-
Thr-Cys-Ala-Lys-Leu-Ser-Gly-Cys-Lys-Ile-Ile-Ser-Gly-Ser-
 25   26   27   28   29   30   31   32   33  34  35  36   37   38
```

Thr-Cys-Pro-Ser-Tyr-Pro-Asx-Lys
Thr-Cys-Pro-Ser-Tyr-Pro-Asp-Lys
 39 40 41 42 43 44 45 46

(Asx means Asp
or Asn)

The position of the disulfide bonds are the same in both proteins. Residue 16 is connected to residue 26 and residues 3 and 4 to residues 32 and 40. However, it is not known at present if residue 3 is linked to residue 32 or to residue 40 and vice versa for residue 4. Viscotoxin B is very like the two other viscotoxins. The main difference seems to be in the sequence of residues 18–25.

Screening of 41 different species of mistletoes for viscotoxin-like proteins has revealed the presence of such substances in 5 species, all within the sub-family Viscoideae. One of these plants, *Phoradendron tomentosum* subsp. *macrophyllum*, has been further investigated and one pure protein, phoratoxin, isolated. Phoratoxin has the same pharmacological effects as the viscotoxins. The molecular weight is around 5000, as determined by ultracentrifugation, and the sequence of the first 4 amino acids is the same as in the viscotoxins.

References

Samuelsson, G. 1961 'Phytochemical and Pharmacological Studies on *Viscum album* L.
   V. Further improvements in the isolation method for Viscotoxin. Studies on
   Viscotoxin from *Viscum album* growing on *Tilia cordata* Mill.' *Svensk Farm
   Tidskr.*, **65**: 481–494.
Samuelsson, G. 1966 'Chromatography of Viscotoxin and oxidized Viscotoxin on phos-
   phate cellulose.' *Acta Chem. Scand.*, **20**: 1546–1554.
Samuelsson, G. and M. Ekblad 1967 'Isolation and properties of phoratoxin, a toxic
   protein from *Phoradendron serotinum* (Loranthaceae).' *Acta. Chem. Scand.*, **21**:
   849–856.
Samuelsson, G. and B. Pettersson 1970 'Separation of viscotoxins from the European
   Mistletoe, *Viscum album* L (Loranthaceae) by chromatography on sulfoethyl
   Sephadex[R].' *Acta Chem. Scand.*, **24**: 2751–2756.
Samuelsson, G., L. Seger and T. Olson 1968 'The amino acid sequence of oxidized
   Viscotoxin A3 from the European Mistletoe (*Viscum album* L., Loranthaceae).'
   Acta Chem. Scand., **22**: 2624–2642.
Rosell, S. and G. Samuelsson 1966 'Effect of Mistletoe Viscotoxin and phoratoxin on
   blood circulation.' *Toxicon*, **4**: 107–110.
Winterfeld, K. and H. Bijl 1948 'Viscotoxin, ein neuer Inhaltstoff der Mistel (*Viscum
   Album* L).' *Ann.*, **561**: 107–115.

TOXIN OF *CLOSTRIDIUM BOTULINUM**

D. A. BOROFF

Laboratory of Research Immunology, Albert Einstein Medical Center
Philadelphia, Pennsylvania, 19141, U.S.A.

ON MOLECULAR BASIS, the toxin of *Clostridium botulinum* is one of the most potent bacterial poisons known. It has been estimated that $10^{-5}\,\mu g$ of the substance contains a minimal lethal dose for a 20 g mouse. The toxin was described in. 1897 by Van Ermengem, who identified it as the etiological agent of the often fatal food poisoning which we know as botulism. The toxin is a neurotoxin (Schubel, 1921) which affects the myoneural junctions of the cholinergic nerve system (Dickson and Shevky, 1923). The action of the toxin has been ascribed to its effect upon the nerve end organs, where it inhibits the release of acetylcholine (Guyton and MacDonald, 1947; Ambache, 1949; Brooks, 1954). There is some evidence, however, that the central nervous system is also involved (Matveev, 1959; Winbury, 1959).

Because of the toxin's exceptional antigenicity and because most of it was usually found in the culture filtrate, this toxin was classed as a typical exotoxin. Raynaud and Second (1949) and Boroff and Raynaud (1952) showed, however, that the toxin could be extracted from the organisms and that upon autolysis the toxin was released into the surrounding medium.

The toxin was isolated and crystallized by Lamanna *et al.* (1946) and independently by Abrams *et al.* in 1946, and was shown to be a simple protein consisting of no unknown amino acids and possessing no unusual grouping to account for its exceptional lethality. It was estimated by these workers that crystalline preparations contained 2×10^8 MLD per mg of

*This investigation is supported in part by National Institutes of Health Grant #ROI-AI04180TOX and National Science Foundation Grant #GB−6719

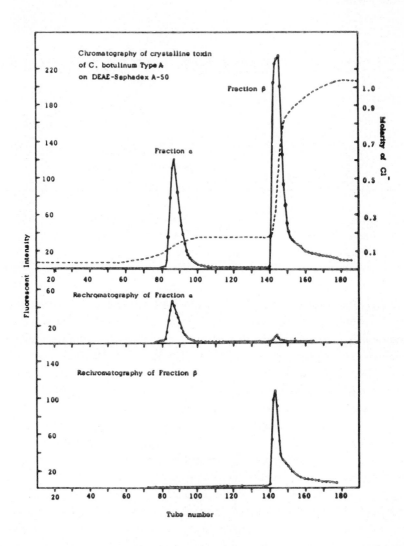

FIGURE 1.   Chromatography of crystalline toxin of *C. botulinum* Type A on DEAE Sephadex. Top section: fractionation of crystalline toxin. Middle section: rechromatography of a portion of pooled α fraction obtained from first run. Bottom section: rechromatography of a portion of pooled β fraction obtained from first run (DasGupta *et al.*, 1966)

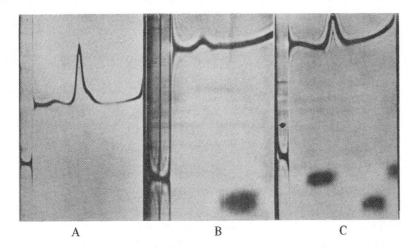

FIGURE 2.   Ultracentrifuge photographs of crystalline toxin and isolated fraction of
C. botulinum Type A at (50700) rpm, 32 minutes after reaching full speed, in 0.05 M
Tris-ClO$_4$, pH 9.5 at 25° C. (A) crystalline toxin; (B) toxic fraction (α); (C) nontoxic

protein nitrogen. The crystalline preparation was thought to be
homogeneous, in spite of the fact that Lamanna and Lowenthal (1951)
observed that the crystals besides being toxic also hemagglutinated red blood
cells. In addition, Wagman (1963) demonstrated that this preparation in the
ultracentrifuge at alkaline pH invariably migrated as two components, one
with 7 and another with 13 to 17 sedimentation velocity coefficients.

The purity of the toxin came into question when it was observed that on
slide immuno-electrophoresis the toxin separated into two distinct
components. The same two components were observed on gel double
diffusion test when anticrystalline toxin serum was placed into the central
well on the Ouchterlony plates. (See Figure 5, well #1.)

The dissociation of the toxin at alkaline pH in the ultracentrifuge served as
a rationale for our attempts to achieve the separation of the two components
on chromatographic columns. Employing DEAE-cellulose columns
equilibrated and eluted with Tris–HCl at pH 8 and a linear gradient of NaCl
we obtained two distinct fractions, one containing ten times the specific
activity of the original material and another only feebly toxic but with strong
hemagglutinating properties (DasGupta and Boroff, 1966) (Figure 1). In the
ultracentrifuge the toxin sedimented with s$_{20}$w value of about 7 and was

calculated to be of 150,000 molecular weight; the second component (β) had $s_{20}w$ of 16, and was of 750,000 molecular weight (Figure 2). The α component appeared to be homogeneous by all criteria applied (Boroff et al., 1966).

End group analysis of α component by Edman degradation method suggested that the N-terminal was blocked. The second stage of degradation yielded enough phenylalanine to indicate the presence of subunits of 60,000 to 90,000 molecular weight. At no time was there evidence present of small molecular weight toxins.

One property of the toxin which attracted our attention was the observation that the toxin fluoresced in the ultra-violet (Boroff and Fitzgerald, 1958). That the toxin fluoresces is not in itself remarkabe. All proteins fluoresce, due to the presence in them of the three aromatic amino acids: tryptophan, tyrosine and phenylalanine. What appeared remarkable was that whenever the fluorescence was destroyed so was the toxicity. The reverse, however, was not true; toxicity could be destroyed without affecting fluorescence (Schantz et al., 1960). Mager, Kindler and Grossowicz (1954) published a series of papers in which they discussed the relationship of amino acids, vitamins and salts to toxin synthesis by *Clostridium botulinum*, and in which they showed the importance of relatively large amounts of tryptophan in toxigenesis. This fact, and the fact that the toxin fluoresced with the wave length of this amino acid directed our attention to its importance in the molecule of the toxin. To investigate the relation of tryptophan to the activity of the toxin we attempted to modify the amino acid by photo-oxidation in visible light in the presence of traces of methylene blue at acid pH (Figure 3). Only tryptophan, methionine and cysteine are affected under these conditions. This treatment destroyed the toxicity and fluorescence and modified the antigenicity of the toxin. The importance of methionine to toxicity was ruled out by the treatment of the toxin with H_2O_2, which specifically modified methionine (Neumann et al., 1962). Destruction of as much as 41.7 moles of methionine out of 62.8 moles of this amino acid per mole of toxin did not significantly affect its activity. Another procedure which modifies tryptophan is treatment with 2 hydroxy-5-nitrobenzyl bromide (HNBB) (Koshland et al., 1964). This reagent modifies tryptophan and cysteine; the effect of the reagent upon the latter is, however, very slow. Treatment of the toxin with HNBB destroyed both the toxicity and the fluorescence (Boroff and DasGupta, 1966). The reaction was instantaneous. Again the antigenicity was modified (Figure 4).

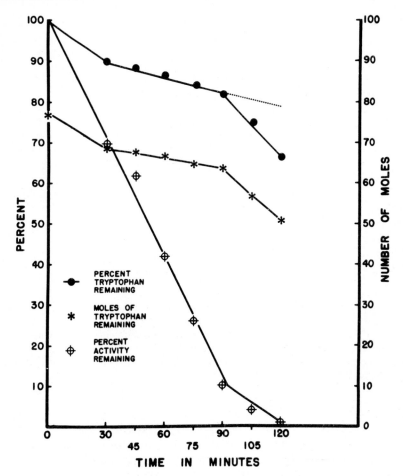

FIGURE 3.   Effect of photooxidation on toxicity and destruction of tryptophan residues in the toxin of *C. botulinum* (Boroff and DasGupta, 1964)

The relation of fluorescence and therefore tryptophan to toxicity was further supported by the observation that when the toxin was combined with its specific antiserum, the toxicity was neutralized and fluorescence reduced. The toxin treated either by photooxidation or by HNBB failed to induce formation of protective antibody when injected into rabbits or to react with crystalline toxin antiserum in serological tests. The hemagglutinin remained unaffected (Figure 5).

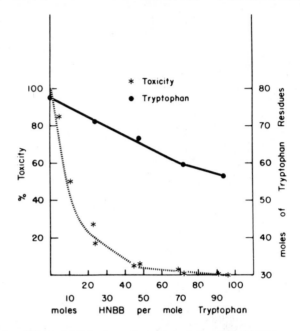

FIGURE 4. Effects of 2 hydroxy-5-nitrobenzyl bromide (HNBB) on toxicity and tryptophan residues of the toxin of *C. botulinum* Type A. Tryptophan assay by Spies and Chambers method. Toxicity assay by intravenous injection in mice (Boroff and DasGupta, 1966)

On the basis of the above observations we postulated that some of the tryptophan residues in the molecule of the toxin were either located in or were contributing to the formation of reactive sites of the toxin.

In titrating the toxin's potency we observed that when toxin is injected intravenously into mice the time of survival of the animals in minutes is inversely proportional to the logarithm of concentration of the toxin. Thus, to double the survival time of the animals the toxin must be diluted ten times (Figure 6). The kinetics of toxin action do not therefore suggest it to be an enzyme. The minuteness of the lethal dose drew attention to the possibility that the toxin might be an antagonist to some substance essential to nerve function. *A priori* such a substance had to be involved in nerve function, present in the body and related to tryptophan. The substance which fulfilled these criteria was serotonin—(5 hydoxy-tryptamine (5HT).) 5HT has been described by Woolley and Gommi (1965) as a neural agent involved in the

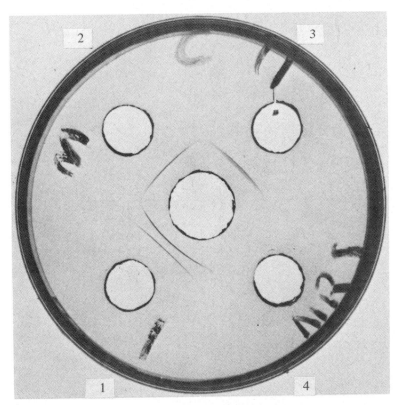

FIGURE 5.   Ouchterlony gel double diffusion test with rabbit antiserum prepared against photooxidized and 5 hydroxy-2-nitrobenzyl bromide treated toxins of *C. botulinum* Type A. Central well contains native crystalline toxin. Well 1, antiserum to native toxin; well 2, photooxidized toxin; well 3, antiserum to 5 hydroxy-2-nitrobenzyl bromide treated toxin; well 4, normal rabbit serum control

transport of calcium through nerve membranes. Calcium was shown to be a releaser of acetylcholine. We reasoned that injection of serotonin should affect the action of the toxin. Indeed, when serotonin was injected intraperitoneally into mice and followed 30 to 60 minutes later by intravenous toxin injection, survival of the mice was significantly prolonged (Table 1). Vasoconstriction, which is among the properties of this substance, was apparently not the factor in prolonging the survival time, since vasopressin injected in sufficient quantities to produce profound vasoconstriction did not noticeably affect survival time of mice.

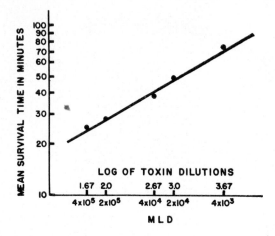

FIGURE 6.   Relation of log of concentration of the toxin of *Clostridium botulinum* to mean survival time of mice

TABLE 1   Effects of time interval between serotonin and botulinum toxin administration on the survival time of mice.

Interval between serotonin and toxin administration[a]	Survival time		MLD[b]
	Range	Average	
Immediately after serotonin	16−18	17	8×10^5
30 min later	32−36.5	35	1.2×10^5
60 min later	39−45	42	6.0×10^4
Toxin alone	24−27	25	3.6×10^5

[a]Crystailine botulinum toxin Type A was injected i.v., 0.1 ml/mouse, and serotonin i.p., 1.0 mg/mouse. Toxin concentration was calculated from standard curve of the relation of toxin concentration to survival time. Six mice were used in each group.
[b]MLD, minimal lethal dose for 20 g albino mice

In summary, the toxin of *Clostridium botulinum* has been isolated as a homogeneous protein of 128,000 to 150,000 molecular weight with possible subunits of 60,000 to 90,000. There is no evidence that the organism produces more than one toxin, or a small molecular weight toxin. The behavior of tryptophan residues in the toxin suggests that it may be located in or is contributing to the formation of reactive sites. The general impression, however, is that the toxin depends upon the integrity of its tertiary structure for its toxic as well as its antigenic activity. The toxin may be an antagonist of some substance essential to nerve function, such as serotonin.

References

Abrams, A., G. Kegeles and G. A. Hottle 1946 'The Purification of toxin from *Clostridium botulinum* Type A.' *J. Biol. Chem.*, **164**: 1.

Ambache, N. 1949 'Peripheral action of botulinum toxin.' *J. Physiol.*, **108**: 127.

Boroff, D. A. and B. R. DasGupta 1966 'Study of the toxin of *C. botulinum*. Effects of 2-hydroxy-5-nitrobenzyl bromide on the biological activity of botulinum toxin.' *Biochim. Biophys. Acta*, **117**: 289.

Boroff, D. A. and J. E. Fitzgerald 1958 'Fluorescence of the toxin of *Clostridium botulinum* and its relation to toxicity.' *Nature*, **181**: 751.

Boroff, D. A. and M. Raynaud 1952 'Studies of toxin of *Clostridium botulinum*, type D.' *J. Immunol.*, **68**: 503.

Boroff, D. A., R. Townhend, U. Fleck and B. R. DasGupta 1966 'Ultracentrifugal analysis of the crystalline toxin and isolated fractions of *Clostridium botulinum* type A.' *J. Biol. Chem.*, **241**: 5165.

Brooks, V. B. 1954 'The action of botulinum toxin on motor nerve filaments.' *J. Physiol.*, **123**: 501.

DasGupta, B. R. *et al.* 1966 'Chromatographic isolation of the crystalline toxin of *Clostridium botulinum* type A.' *Biochem. Biophys. Res. Comm.*, **22**: 750.

Dickson, E. C. and C. Shevky 1923 'Botulism studies on the manner in which the toxin of *Clostridium botulinum* acts on the body. I. The effects on the autonomic nervous system.' *J. Exptl. Med.*, **37**: 711.

Guyton, A. C. and M. A. McDonald 1947 'Physiology of botulinum toxin.' *Arch. Neurol. Psychiat.*, **57**: 578.

Koshland, D. E., V. D. Karkhanis and M. G. Latham 1964 'An environmentally-sensitive reagent with selectivity for the tryptophan residue in proteins.' *J. Amer. Chem. Soc.*, **86**: 1448.

Lamanna, C. and J. P. Lowenthal 1951 'The lack of identity between hemagglutinin and the toxin of type A botulinal toxin.' *J. Bacteriol.*, **61**: 751.

Lamanna, C., D. E. McElroy and H. W. Eklund 1946 'The purification and crystallization of *Clostridium botulinum*, type A Toxin.' *Science*, **103**: 613.

Mager, J., S. H. Kindler and N. Grossowicz 1954 'Nutritional studies with *Clostridium parabotulinum* type A.' *J. Gen. Microbiol.*, **10**: 130.

Matveev, K. I. 1959 '*Botulism*, Monograph.' Moscow State Publishers of Medical Literature, Moscow, 179.

Neumann, N. P., S. Moore and W. M. Stein 1962 'Modification of methionin residues in ribonuclease.' *Biochemistry*, **1**: 68.

Raynaud, M. and L. Second 1949 'Extraction des toxines botuliniques a partir des corps microbiens.' *Ann. Inst. Pasteur (Paris)*, **77**: 316.

Schantz, E. J., D. Stefanye and L. Spero 1960 'Observations on the fluorescence and toxicity of botulinum toxin.' *J. Biol. Chem.*, **235**: 3489.

Schubel, K. 1921 'Uber das Botulinus Toxin.' *Deutsch. Med. Wschr.* (Stuttgart), **47**: 1047.

Wagman, J. 1963 'Low molecular weight forms of type A botulinum toxin. II. Action of pepsin on intact and dissociated toxin.' *Arch. Biochem.*, **100**: 414.

Winbury, M. M. 1959 'Mechanism of the local vascular actions.' *J. Physiol.*, **147**: 1.

Woolley, D. W. and B. W. Gommi 1965 'Serotonin receptors. VI. Methods for the direct measurement of isolated receptors.' *Proc. Nat. Acad. Sci.*, **53**: 959.

PHARMACOLOGY

THE BIOCHEMISTRY AND PHARMACOLOGY OF SNAKE VENOMS

F. E. RUSSELL

Laboratory of Neurological Research, Los Angeles County,
University of Southern California Medical Center, Los Angeles,
California, U.S.A.

FEW GROUPS of substances are as complex and varied in their composition and as complicated and diversified in their modes of actions as the snake venoms. It appears that snake poisons are mixtures of 10 to 25 different substances, most of which are proteins or peptides. There was a time in our thinking, and this was not so many years ago, when all of the deleterious pharmacological effects of snake venoms were attributed to the enzymes of the venom. This is easy to understand, for the progress in the methods of enzyme identification had advanced far beyond those for identification of the peptides and proteins of low molecular weight. Thus, it was not unusual for an investigator to seek to explain all of the biological activities of a snake venom on the basis of the presence of some enzyme or combination of enzymes.

With the initial contributions of Wieland and Konz (1936), Ghosh and De (1937), Micheel *et al.* (1937), Slotta and Frankel-Conrat (1938), Ghosh *et al.* (1941), and others, it became evident that there were several nonenzymatic proteins in snake venoms that possessed important biological activities. Although the early separations were far from pure they provided the impetus for the design of more definitive experiments and, indeed, stimulated the interest which subsequently gave rise to the contributions of Neumann and Habermann (1955), Gonçalves (1956), Habermann (1957), Sasaki (1957), Detrait and Boquet (1958), and others.

By the beginning of the last decade, studies on the snake venom peptides and polypeptides were in progress in at least a dozen institutions. If I can be forgiven for errors of commission and ommission in this short review, I should like to note but a few of these more recent works. At the first *International Symposium on Animal Toxins* in April of 1966, Tamiya (1966) presented a paper on the chromatography, crystallization, ultracentrifugation and amino acid analysis of the venom of the sea snake *Laticauda semifasciata*. On CM-cellulose chromatography, 100% of the lethal fraction was recovered as pure erabutoxin *a* and *b*. Thirty per cent of the proteins of the original venom were erabutoxins. The homogeneity of the crystalline toxins was demonstrated by rechromatography, disc electrophoresis and ultracentrifugation. Erabutoxin *b* was more basic than *a*. This was explained by the differences in basic amino acid content, assuming most of the acidic amino acids were in their amido form. Sixty-one amino acids were found in each of the toxins; no alanine or methionine was present. One of the three arginine residues in erabutoxin was at the *N*-terminus. The crystals demonstrated by these workers were thought to be sulfate salts of the basic toxins. The molecular weight of erabutoxin *a* was 6,760 and erabutoxin *b* 6,780 (Tamiya *et al.*, 1967).

Karlsson *et al.* (1966), using ion-exchange chromatography on Amberlite IRC-50, isolated a 'neurotoxin' (toxin α) from *Naja nigricollis* venom which was approximately 3% of the total weight of the crude venom. It was homogeneous by chromatography, free zone electrophoresis, starch gel electrophoresis, immunoelectrophoresis, and end-group analysis. It contained 61 amino acids in a single chain cross-linked by four disulfide bridges and terminated by leucine and asparagine at its amino- and carboxyl- terminal ends. The formula weight was 6,787. The intravenous LD_{100} in 18–20 g mice was 1.8 μg, or approximately 1/9 that of the crude venom.

In 1967, Moroz *et al.*, using ion exchange chromatography and differential salt precipitation, found that the neurotoxin of *Vipera palestinae* venom had a molecular weight of 11,600. The toxin was homogeneous on ultracentrifugation and electrophoresis, and by immunological criteria. It contained 108 amino acid residues.

Larsen and Wolff (1968) isolated two basic proteins, cobramine A and B, by carboxymethyl cellulose chromotography, gel filtration and ammonium sulfate crystallization from the venom of *Naja naja*. The molecular weight of cobramine B was 6,400 on the basis of equilibrium centrifugation and 5,840 on the basis of amino acid analysis.

Yang *et al.* (1969), on the basis of amino acid composition, have calculated the cobratoxin of *Naja naja atra* venom to have a minimum molecular weight of 6,949. Sato *et al.* (1969) have isolated a 'neurotoxic' protein from the venom of *Laticauda laticaudata* and *L. colubrina* with a molecular weight of 6,520. Botes and Strydom (1969) have isolated a 'neurotoxin' from the venom of *Naja haje*, while Dubnóff and Russell (1970) have isolated a protein and two peptides with interesting pharmacological properties from the venom of *Crotalus viridis helleri*. The former has a molecular weight of approximately 30,000, while the two peptides have weights of about 6,000 each.

These and other recent studies indicate the small molecular size of some of the more deleterious fractions of snake venoms. The pharmacological properties of these substances have not yet been fully established. Most of these peptides or small proteins have been called 'neurotoxins', and it would appear that their most obvious property is directed toward the nervous system, but it must be admitted that at the present time few of the other possible pharmacological properties of these peptides have been examined. It has often occurred to this writer that when these toxins evolved, adapted or developed, they may have done so with more relationship to their biological significance and function than to the convenience of man's gobbledegook systems of classification. I have yet to find a 'neurotoxin' in snake venoms which did not have important pharmacological effects on cells or organs other than the nervous system. How often have some of us pleaded that it is more important to tell precisely what a venom or venom fraction does rather than to put a tag—'neurotoxin', 'hemotoxin', or 'cardiotoxin'—on it for the sake of convenience (Russell, 1962).

As already noted, the work on the enzymes of snake venoms has greatly overshadowed that on the non-enzymatic components of this poison. Even today, some 40 articles on snake venom enzymes are published for every one on non-enzymes. Our knowledge on these enzymes is rather respectable, as one might surmise from the fact that almost 800 articles have been written on these substances and their properties (Russell and Scharfenberg, 1964, and updating 1964–69). Certainly, the fine works of Tsuchiya (1936), Slotta (1938), Iyengar (1938), Ghosh (1941), and Zeller (1948), initiated great interest in these proteins, and this interest has not abated during the past two decades.

Table 1 shows some of the more important enzymes found in snake venoms. Space does not permit my attempting to organize these according to their presence in the various families of snakes, but I have noted this else-

TABLE 1   Some enzymes of snake venoms

Proteinases	Desoxyribonuclease
Transaminase	Phosphomonoesterase
Hyaluronidase	Phosphodiesterase
L-Amino acid oxidase	5'-Nucleotidase
Cholinesterase	ATPase
Phospholipase A	DPNase
Phospholipase B and C	Endonucleases
Ribonuclease	

References cited in Russell (1967b)

where (Russell, 1967a; 1967b), and at this time I should only like to consider some of the more important biological effects of these enzymes.

Proteinases have been found in most of the snake venoms. All Crotalidae venoms so far examined appear to be rich in proteolytic enzyme activity. The Viperidae venoms have lesser amounts, while the Elapidae and Hydrophiidae venoms either have no proteolytic enzyme activity or very little. There does not appear to be a pattern or relationship between the various crotalid and viperid genera and the amount of proteinase present in their venoms. Venoms that are rich in proteinase produce marked tissue changes and destruction. What role this enzyme may play in the deleterious blood changes produced by some snake venoms is still unresolved. The anticoagulant effect of several reptile venoms may be due in part to the proteolytic disintegration of fibrinogen. The coagulant effect of other venoms may also be due in part to the formation of thrombin from prothrombin, a change catalyzed by certain proteinases.

Hyaluronidase has been found in every snake venom so far examined. It hydrolyzes the hyaluronic acid gel of the spaces between cells and fibers, particularly in connective tissue, and thus reduces the viscosity of these tissues. This breakdown in the hyaluronic acid barrier allows other fractions of the venom to penetrate the tissues. The enzyme is obviously related to the extent of the edema and swelling caused by snake venoms, but to what degree it contributes to these signs is not known.

L-Amino acid oxidase has been found in over 70 snake venoms. It catalyzes the oxidation of L-α-amino acids and of α-hydroxy acids. It is the most active of the known amino acid oxidases, and ophio-L-amino acid oxidase is probably a group of homologous enzymes.

Few enzymes are as capable of attacking so many different substances as L-amino acid oxidase. Zeller (1951) suggests that the enzyme is probably not a toxic component of snake venoms, but that its action is integrated with the digestive function of the venom. If this oxidase is responsible for the activating power of snake venoms it may be considered as a nonhydrolytic digestive enzyme. As Zeller has noted, the enzyme is not present in venoms obtained from organs which are not developed from digestive glands, such as those of the bee and scorpion. We have not found this enzyme in 8 species of scorpions, 9 species of venomous fishes or 2 species of poisonous fishes. The data from spiders are inconclusive.

The L-amino acid oxidase from the venom of *Vipera ammodytes* has been purified by selective heat denaturation, zone electrophoresis, chromatography and by other means (Zwisler, 1965).

The ophio-L-amino acid oxidase of *Crotalus* venom does not contribute to the profound fall in systemic arterial pressure produced by the crude venom following its intravenous injection into mammals. It does not have a deleterious effect on neuromuscular transmission. While its intravenous LD_{50} in mice was found to be 9.13 mg. per kilogram body weight, it may be that this effect was due to the presence of a nonenzymatic venom component separated with the oxidase. However, even if the enzyme was pure, this LD_{50} might not be significant if one considers that in the particular venom studied the enzyme accounted for less than 3 per cent of the total weight of the crude venom; thus the oxidase would contribute to less than 1 per cent of the total lethality of the venom. It is also interesting to note that the antivenin prepared against this venom neutralized the lethal effect of the L-amino acid oxidase studied (Russell *et al.*, 1963).

Cholinesterase has been identified in the venoms of at least 50 snakes. As a whole, elapid venoms are rich in the enzyme, while viperid and crotalid venoms either do not contain the enzyme or possess it in only small amounts. The enzyme catalyzes the hydrolysis of acetylcholine to choline and acetic acid. A number of workers have shown the enzyme to be an acetylcholinesterase. In normal tissues the enzyme prevents the excessive accumulation of acetylcholine at cholinergic synapses and at the neuromuscular junction, among other activities.

As the earlier studies on elapid venoms showed the marked effects of these venoms on neuromuscular activity, and as these venoms contained large amounts of cholinesterase, it was thought that the enzyme was responsible for the curare-like effect of the whole venom and the death of the animal. It is now known that cholinesterase plays a relatively insignificant role in the neuromuscular blocking phenomenon produced by elapid venoms. What part this enzyme plays in the over-all effect of the crude venom is not known. It is known that some venoms free of the enzyme increase the cholinesterase activity of intact squid nerve, possibly by altering permeability and thus allowing an access of substrate (Rosenberg and Dettbarn, 1964).

Phospholipase A, B, C, and D are catalysts involved in the hydrolysis of lipids. Snake venom phospholipase A catalyzes the hydrolysis of one of the fatty ester linkages in diacyl phosphatides, forming lysophosphatidase and releasing both saturated and unsaturated fatty acids. Some snake venoms may contain several enzymes with phospholipase A activity. Saito and Hanahan (1962) isolated two phospholipases with molecular weights of approximately 30,000 to 35,000 and isoelectric points of pH 4.40 and 5.55 from the venom of the rattlesnake *Crotalus adamanteus*.

It is generally thought that the hemolysis produced by snake venoms is due to the action of phospholipase A. This may be due to a direct action in which the phospholipids of the red cell membrane are hydrolyzed, or it may be due to an indirect action through the production of lysolecithin from plasma lecithin by the phospholipase. Direct lytic venoms, such as those of certain Australian elapids, produce intravascular hemolysis; while indirect lytic venoms, which produce marked *in vitro* and *in vivo* changes in red cells, may produce intravascular hemolysis. However, such hemolysis is influenced or perhaps determined by other factors, such as the plasma lecithin level, the protective effect of the plasma proteins, the possible sensitivity of the red cells to lysolecithin, and the influence of the spleen.

Venom phospholipase A is known to release histamine from the rat diaphragm, and a slow-reacting substance which produces hemolysis from certain other tissues. It probably plays some role in disrupting the normal sequence of electron transfer by phospholipids.

The role of phospholipase A in altering nerve, muscle, or neuromuscular junction conduction and possible central nervous system activity is a consideration that has elicited much controversy. Certainly, its ability to destroy or alter certain phospholipids in nerve tissues essential to electron transfer could make it a neurotoxin. It has been claimed by some workers that this enzyme is the neurotoxic component of snake venoms but this seems unlikely. It may contribute to a neurotoxic effect by its action on phospholipids in nerve tissues, but it is hardly responsible for the more severe and more rapid pharmacological changes provoked by the crude venom in nerve tissues. It is quite possible that venom phospholipase A facilitates the penetration of neuropharmacologically active venom components into nerve tissue and in this way contributes to the neurological deficit.

Phospholipase B catalyzes the hydrolysis of lysolecithin to glycerophosphocholine and fatty acid. It has been found in the venom of a number of snakes. Phospholipase C catalyzes the hydrolysis of phosphatidylcholine to a diglyceride and choline phosphate. The pharmacological effects of these two enzymes from snake venom are not known.

Snake venoms contain several phosphatases involved in the hydrolysis of phosphate bonds in nucleotides. These are phosphomonoesterase, phosphodiesterase, 5'-nucleotidase, ATPase, DPNase, and endonuclease.

Phosphomonoesterase has properties of an orthophosphoric monoester phosphohydrolase. Nothing is known about the pharmacological properties of venom phosphomonoesterase.

Phosphodiesterase has been found in almost all snake venoms tested. It is an orthophosphoric diester phosphohydrolase which also releases 5-nucleotides from polynucleotides, thus acting as an exonucleotidase. It has been suggested that the enzyme is responsible for the ATPase and DPNase activities of venoms.

Phosphodiesterase prepared after the method of Williams, Sung, and Laskowski (1960) produces an immediate and profound fall in the systemic arterial pressure of cats after its intravenous injection. In mice, its intravenous LD_{50} was found to be approximately 4.0 mg per kilogram body weight; it produced no deleterious changes in nerve-muscle conduction in the mammal (Russell *et al.*, 1963). These actions, while they may be due to the enzyme, might also be caused by some other substance separated with the enzyme, since on disc electrophoresis the same phosphodiesterase was shown to be composed of several fractions.

5'-Nucleotidase is a common constituent of all snake venoms. In most instances it is the most active phosphatase in the venom. It is a 5'-ribonucleotide phosphohydrolase which catalyzes the hydrolysis of 5'-mononucleotides, yielding the ribonucleoside and orthophosphate.

Maeno and Mitsuhashi (1961) identified at least three 5'-nucleotidase fractions on chromatography, two of which were associated with lethal activity. Master and Rao (1963) also separated the enzyme from a toxic component. It seems likely, however, that the electrophoretic mobility of the enzyme is the same as that of the unidentified lethal fraction, as the latter authors have noted.

Acetylcholine is present in large amounts in *Dendroaspis* venoms and in small amounts in *Naja, Crotalus, Sistrurus,* and *Agkistrodon* venoms. None has been found in the venoms of *Bungarus, Hemachatus, Pseudechis, Vipera, Bitis,* or *Bothrops.* Welsh (1967) suggests that in *Dendroaspis*, its role might be in the defense armament, or it may act directly on the heart or at the neuromuscular junction of the prey. It may possibly facilitate the distribution of the more toxic components of the venom.

It is easy to see that the sites of action of a snake venom may be, and usually are, multiple, and this indicates again the care that must be taken in labelling a venom as a neurotoxin, hemotoxin, or cardiotoxin. *Crotalus* venoms, for instance, provoke deleterious local tissue changes, changes in the dynamics of the heart; in the resistance and permeability of the blood vessels, particularly in those of the pulmonary system; in the integrity and viscosity of the blood cells; in conduction along nerves, at the neuromuscular junction, at the muscle, or in the central nervous system or spinal cord; and changes in the respiratory system at various levels.

In clinical cases, *Crotalus* venom causes swelling, edema, ecchymosis, and tissue changes leading to necrosis and, in some cases, sloughing at the area of envenomation. The venom alters the permeability of the blood vessels, and this leads to loss of plasma, and in many cases loss of blood, into the tissues. This is manifested by ecchymosis and, in more severe cases hematuria, melena, hematemesis, epistaxis, and hemoptysis. Bleeding, coagulation, and prothrombin times are increased. The red blood cells undergo changes which are first evident by their swelling and sphering. The hematocrit may fall rapidly, and platelets may all but disappear from the smear. Pulmonary edema is common in the more severe cases, and bleeding phenomena may occur in the lungs, peritoneum, kidneys, and heart. These changes are often accompanied by alterations in cardiac dynamics and renal function.

However, not all *Crotalus* venoms produce this picture. The venom of the Mojave rattlesnake, *Crotalus scutulatus scutulatus*, produces far less tissue destruction but far greater changes in conduction, particularly in neuromuscular transmission. In this respect it is similar to that of the tropical rattlesnake *Crotalus durissus terrificus*.

The mechanisms of these various changes have been studied in some detail. In most cases of rattlesnake venom poisoning, the clinical picture follows that noted above. But in an occasional case, and in experiments with laboratory animals, death occurs rather rapidly and the mechanism of death in these cases has been of considerable interest to pharmacologists. In such cases, there is an immediate and profound fall in systemic arterial pressure. This does not appear to be due to a decrease in heart rate or contractile force, although even small amounts of venom may elicit cardiac depression. It is not due to a deficit in venous return, depression of the central nervous system, sudden electrolytic imbalance, or a decrease in total blood volume. There is, however, a marked fall in circulating blood volume, which appears to be due to pooling.

In our own studies in cats and in certain observations on humans, the pooling has occurred in the major blood vessels of the chest and in the lungs. The pooling was evident in the capillary bed; and simultaneous measurements in cats and monkeys of pulmonary artery pressure and flow, the pressure in the left atrium, and certain other parameters suggested that the first recordable changes in blood dynamics were due to an increase in resistances in the post-capillary veins, possibly in the smaller venules (Russell *et al.*, 1962). Following this, there was an increase in lung capillary blood with a resulting increase in pulmonary artery pressure and a decrease in pulmonary artery flow. Cardiac pressures were related to this change, as were peripheral systemic arterial and venous pressures. In cases where blood transfusions or intravenous fluids were given immediately following this hypotensive crisis, the per cent of survivals was increased. In those cases where death occurred, there was sludging and clumping of erythrocytes, formation of thrombi, particularly in the lungs and pulmonary circuit, petechial hemorrhages in the lungs (which might be attributed to the increased capillary bed flooding and increased pressure, as well as to the direct effect of the venom on the vessel walls), and the formation of thromboemboli. Once these phenomena had developed, only the use of renal dialysis, exchange transfusions and antivenin prolonged life, but in most experiments they did not change the mortality rate, probably because irreversible damage to the heart, lungs and kidneys had already been done.

In conclusion, it might be said that our knowledge of the chemistry and pharmacology of snake venoms and their fractions, and of the autopharmacological response to these toxins, is comforting but far from complete. Numerous laboratories are now working on the specific modes of action of specific venom fractions. The data derived from these studies has already contributed to more effective therapeutic measures, to the production of hyperantivenins, to the development of new medicines, and perhaps, the most important contribution of all, to the use of venom fractions as tools in biology for the study of cellular structure and function.

SUMMARY

The author discusses the present state of knowledge on the chemistry and pharmacology of snake venoms, and reviews the important investigations that have led up to the definitive studies now being done.

References

Botes, D. P. and D. J. Strydom 1969 'A neurotoxin, toxin α, from Egyptian cobra (*Naja haje haje*) venom. I. Purification, properties and complete amino acid sequence.' *J. Biol. Chem.*, **244**: 4147.

Detrait, J. and P. Boquet 1958 'Separation des constituants du venin de *Naja naja* par l'electrophorèse.' *Compt. Rend. Acad. Sci. D.*, **246**: 1107.

Dubnoff, J. W. and F. E. Russell 1970 'Isolation of a lethal protein and peptide from *Crotalus viridis helleri* venom.' *Proc. Western Pharmac. Soc.* **13**: 98

Ghosh, B. N. and S. S. De 1937 'The migration of the toxic constituents of cobra (*Naja naja*) venom at various pH in an electric field.' *Indian J. Med. Res.*, **24**: 1175.

Ghosh, B. N., S. S. De and D. K. Chowdhury 1941a 'Separation of the neurotoxin from the crude venom and study of the action of a number of reducing agents on it.' *Indian J. Med. Res.*, **29**: 367.

Ghosh, B. N., S. S. De and D. K. Chowdhury 1941b 'Enzymes in snake venom.' *Ann. Biochem.*, **1**: 31.

Gonçalves, J. M. 1956 'Purification and properties of crotamine.' *In*: Buckley, E. E. and N. Porges (eds.), *Venoms*, p. 261. American Association for the Advancement of Science, Washington, D. C.

Habermann, E. 1957 'Gewinnung und Eigenschaften von Crotactin, Phospholipase A, Crotamin und "Toxin III" aus dem Gift der brasilianischen Klapperschlange.' *Biochem. Z.*, **329**: 405.

Iyengar, K. B., K. B. Sehra, B. Mukerji and R. N. Chopra 1938 'Cholinesterase in cobra venom.' *Curr. Sci. India*, **7**: 51.

Karlsson, E., D. L. Eaker and J. Porath 1966 'Purification of a neurotoxin from the venom of *Naja nigricollis*.' *Biochim. Biophys. Acta*, **127**: 505.

Larsen, P. R. and J. Wolff 1968 'The basic proteins of cobra venom. I. Isolation and characterization of cobramines A and B.' *J. Biol. Chem.*, **243**: 1283.

Maeno, H. and S. Mitsuhashi 1961 'Studies on Habu snake venom. IV. Fractionation of Habu snake venom by chromatography on CM cellulose.' *J. Biochem.*, **50**: 434.

Master, R. W. P. and S. S. Rao 1963 'Starch gel electrophoresis of venoms of Indian krait and saw-scaled viper and identification of enzymes and toxins.' *Biochim. Biophys. Acta*, **71**: 416.

Micheel, F., H. Dietrich and G. Bischoff 1937 'Über die Neurotoxine aus Giften von Cobra-arten.' *Z. Physiol. Chem.*, **249**: 157.

Moroz, C., L. Grotto, N. Goldblum and A. de Vries 1967 'Enhancement of immuno-genicity of snake venom neurotoxins.' *In*: Russell, F. E. and P. R. Saunders (eds.), *Animal Toxins*, p. 299. Pergamon Press, Oxford.

Neumann, W. P. and E. Habermann 1955 'Über Crotactin, das Haupttoxin des Giftes der brasilianischen Klapperschlange (*Crotalus terrificus terrificus*).' *Biochem. Z.*, **327**: 170.

Rosenberg, P. and W. D. Dettbarn 1964 'Increased cholinesterase activity of intact cells caused by snake venoms.' *Biochem. Pharmacol.*, **13**: 1157.

Russell, F. E. 1962 'Snake venom poisoning.' *In*: Piersol, G. M. (ed.), *Cyclopedia of Medicine, Surgery and the Specialities*. Vol. II, p. 199. F. A. Davis Company, Philadelphia.

Russell, F. E. 1967a 'Pharmacology of animal venoms.' *Clin. Pharmacol. Therap.*, **8**: 849.

Russell, F. E. 1967b 'Comparative pharmacology of some animal toxins.' *Federation Proc.*, **26**: 1206.

Russell, F. E. and R. S. Scharffenberg 1964 *Bibliography of Snake Venoms and Venomous Snakes.* Bibliographic Associates, West Covina, California. (Up-dated to 1969).

Russell, F. E., F. W. Buess and J. Strassberg 1962 'Cardiovascular response in *Crotalus* venom.' *Toxicon*, 1: 5.

Russell, F. E., F. W. Buess, M. Y. Woo and R. Eventov 1963a 'Zootoxicological properties of venom L-amino acid oxidase.' *Toxicon*, 1: 229.

Russell, F. E., F. W. Buess, and M. Y. Woo 1963b 'Zootoxicological properties of venom phosphodiesterase.' *Toxicon*, 1: 99.

Saito, K. and D. J. Hanahan 1962 'A study of the purification and properties of the phospholipase A on *Crotalus adamanteus* venom.' *Biochemistry*, 1: 521.

Sasaki, T. 1957 'Chemical studies on the poison of Formosan cobra. II. The terminal amino acid residues of purified poison (neurotoxin).' *J. Pharmacol. Soc. Japan.*, 77: 845.

Sato, S., H. Yoshida, H. Abe and N. Tamiya 1969 'Properties and biosynthesis of a neurotoxic protein of the venoms of sea snakes *Laticauda laticaudata* and *Laticauda colubrina.*' *Biochem. J.*, 115: 85.

Slotta, K. H. 1938 'A crotoxina, primeira substancia pura dos veneos ofidicos.' *Ann. Acad. Bras. Sci.*, 10: 195.

Slotta, K. and H. Fraenkel-Conrat 1938 'Two active proteins from rattlesnake venom.' *Nature*, 142: 213.

Tamiya, N., H. Arai and S. Sato 1967 'Studies on sea snake venoms: Crystallization of erabutoxins "a" and "b" from *Laticauda semifasciata* venom.' *In*: Russell, F. E. and P. R. Saunders (eds.), *Animal Toxins*. p. 249. Pergamon Press, Oxford.

Tsuchiya, Y. 1936 'Enzyme chemical investigation of Formosan snake venoms. IV. Activation of peptidase by the snake venoms. 6. Absorption and elution of the active constituent of the venom of *Naja naja atra* Cantor.' *Mem. Fac. Sci. Agric. Taihoku*, 9: 309.

Welsh, J. H. 1967 'Acetylcholine in snake venoms.' *In*: Russell, F. E. and P. R. Saunders (eds.), *Animal Toxins*, p. 363. Pergamon Press, Oxford.

Wieland, H., and W. Konz 1936 *'Einige Beobachtungen am Gift der Brillenschlangen (Naja tripudians).* Sitzungber.' Bayerische Akad. Wiss. Math.-Naturwiss. Abteil. p. 177.

Williams, E. J., S. C. Sung and M. Laskowski 1960 'Action of venom phosphodiesterase on deoxyribonucleic acid.' *J. Biol. Chem.*, 236: 1130.

Yang, C. C., C. C. Chang, K. Hayashi and T. Suzuki 1969 'Amino acid composition and end group analysis of cobratoxin.' *Toxicon*, 7: 43.

Zeller, E. A. 1948 'Enzymes of snake venoms and their biological significance.' *In*: Nord, F. F. (ed.), *Advances in Enzymology*, Vol. 8, p. 459. Interscience Publishers, Inc., New York.

Zeller, E. A. 1951 'Enzymes as essential components of bacterial and animal toxins.' *In*: Sumner, J. B. and K. Myrback (eds.), *The Enzymes*. p. 986. Academic Press, New York.

Zwisler, O. 1965 'Über L-aminosäureoxydase aus Gift der *Vipera ammodytes.*' *Z. Physiol. Chem.*, 343: 178.

ACTIONS NEUROMUSCULAIRES DE FRACTIONS ISOLEES DE VENINS DE SERPENTS

J. CHEYMOL, F. BOURILLET ET M. ROCH-ARVEILLER

Instituté de Pharmacologie, Faculté de Médecine de Paris,
Paris, France

NOUS NOUS SOMMES CONSACRES depuis quelques années à l'étude des effets neuromusculaires de plusieurs venins de serpents appartenant à diverses familles ophidiennes (Tableau 1).

L'action des venins est le plus souvent complexe. Ce sont, en effet, des mélanges de diverses fractions protidiques plus ou moins actives ou toxiques. L'action de ces venins correspond à la superposition des effets de chacune des fractions qu'il faut étudier séparément après purification, si on veut analyser chacun des mécanismes en jeu.

Certaines toxines ont pu être isolées et analysées. Nous rapportons ici les résultats obtenus avec quatre d'entre elles de nature polypeptidique dont la pureté a été vérifiée par immunoélectrophorèse:

La toxine α du venin de *Naja nigricollis* isolée par le Dr. P. Boquet (Boquet *et al.*, 1966; Karlsson *et al.*, 1966); les Erabutoxines a et b isolées du venin de *Laticauda semifasciata* par le Pr. N. Tamiya (Tamiya et Arai, 1966; Tamiya *et al.*, 1967); la Crotamine isolée du venin de *Crotalus durissus terrificus* var. *crotaminicus* par le Pr. J. Moura Gonçalves (Gonçalves, 1956; Gonçalves et Giglio, 1964).

CROTAMINE

C'est une fraction polypeptidique isolée du venin de *Crotalus durissus*

TABLEAU 1   Effets de venins de diverses familles ophidiennes

	FAMILLE	VENINS ETUDIÉS	ACTION du VENIN	TOXINES ETUDIEES
PROTEROGLYPHES	ELAPIDAE	*Naja naja* *Naja nigricollis* *Naje haje* *Hemachatus haemachatus*	paralysant et cardiotoxique	Toxine α (Boquet *et al.*, 1966)
	HYDROPHIIDAE	*Lapemis hardwickii* *Hydrophis cyanocinctus* *Enhydrina schistosa* *Laticauda semifasciata*	paralysant	Erabutoxine a Erabutoxine b (Tamiya *et al.*, 1967)
SOLENOGLYPHES	CROTALIDAE	*Crotalus durissus* *terrificus* variété sans crotamine à crotamine	paralysant contracturant	Crotamine (Gonçalves, 1964)
		Bothrops atrox *B. jararaca* *B. lanceolatus* *B. carribaeus*	aucun effet neuromusculaire mais coagulant, et nécrosant.	

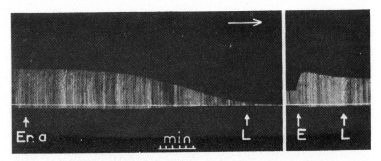

FIGURE 7.   Diaphragme isolé de Rat.
En ↑ Er. a-addition au bain de 2 μg/ml d'érabutoxine a;
En L-lavage;
En ↑ E (t + 2h 48 min) 16 μg/ml d'édrophonium

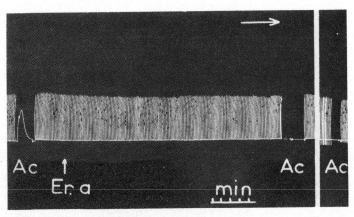

FIGURE 8.   Diaphragme de Rat chroniquement dénervé.
En Ac (t = 0, t + 1h, t + 2h) 1 μg/ml d'acetylcholine;
En ↑ Er. a–0.75 μg/ml d'érabutoxine a pendant 1 heure

sont lentement bloqués de façon plus ou moins irréversible selon les toxines: ce blocage ressemble à une véritable curarisation. Il peut être démontré par quelques expériences empruntées à l'une ou l'autre de ces toxines: antagonisme de la contracture acetylcholinique sur diaphragme dénervé isolé (Figure 8); sensibilisation à la *d*-tubocurarine; antagonisme partiel de la paralysie par néostigmine et édrophonium (Figure 9).

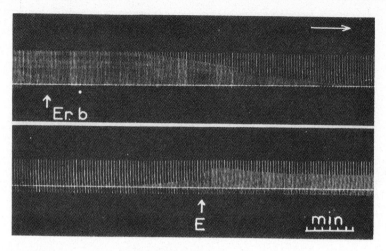

FIGURE 9.   Stimulation directe et indirecte alternée du tibial antérieur *in situ*
En ↑ Er. b = injection i/v de 150 µg/kg d'érabutoxine b;
En ↑ E (t + 5h 10) édrophonium 500 µg/kg i/v

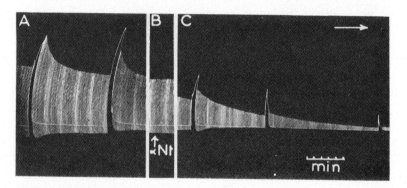

FIGURE 10.   Diaphragme isolé de Rat.
En A: t = 0 stimulation 10 c/sec 30 sec;
        t + 10 min stimulation 50 c/sec 30 sec;
En B: t + 30 ↑ α Nt—addition 1 µg/ml najatoxine;
En C: t + 1h: 10 c/sec 30 sec;
        t + 1h 10: 50 c/sec 30 sec;
        t + 1h 25: 50 c/sec 30 sec

TABLEAU 2   Composition en acides amines de diverses toxines de venins de serpents

	Najatoxine α	Erabutoxine 'a'	Erabutoxine 'b'	Laticotoxine 'a'	Crotamine
ASP	7	5	4	9	3
THR	8	5	5	4	0
SER	2	8	8	5	3
GLU	6	8	8	7	2
PRO	5	4	4	5	4
GLY	5	5	5	5	5
ALA	0	0	0	0	0
CYS ½	8	8	8	8	4
VAL	2	2	2	1	0
MET	0	0	0	0	1
ILE	3	4	4	2	1
LEU	2	1	1	1	1
TYR	1	1	1	1	1
PHE	0	2	2	1	2
LYS	6	4	4	4	11
HIS	2	1	2	2	3
ARG	3	3	3	5	2
TRY	1	1	1	1	3
Total AA	61	62	62	61	46
PM minimal	6,787	6,837	6,857	6,880	5,450

Un autre fait expérimental obtenu avec ces toxines diffère de la curarisation: la tenue d'un tétanos. Après *d*-tubocurarine, le tétanos n'est pas tenu; avec l'α Najatoxine le tétanos est au contraire bien tenu même si la paralysie est profonde (Figure 10).

CONCLUSION

Quels rapprochements peut-on faire entre l'activité neuromusculaire et la constitution de ces toxines?

Ce sont des chaînes polypeptidiques nettement basiques, caractère indispensable à un tropisme neuromusculaire.

Le Tableau 2 montre que la crotamine est constituée de 46 acides aminés avec un poids moléculaire de 5,450. Les autres toxines -y compris la laticotoxine étudiée par Tamiya (1967) sont toutes paralysantes et sont formées de 61 ou 62 acides aminés avec un poids moléculaire (PM) voisin de 6,800. Ce poids moléculaire élevé peut expliquer la différence de cinétique entre ces toxines et la d-tubocurarine (PM 785)—latence, action prolongée, par la difficulté d'atteindre les récepteurs et de s'en séparer spontanément ou sous l'effet d'antagonistes (néostigmine—édrophonium) de faible poids moléculaire.

La composition en acides aminés présente un certain nombre de parallélismes et en particulier la présence dans toutes les toxines de 8 restes hémicystine dont le rôle particulier est de fixer la structure spatiale de la chaine peptidique par les ponts disulfure qu'ils forment: cette chaîne est en effet repliée sur elle-même, pelotonnée; la molécule a donc une structure massive rappelant les pachycurares plutôt que les leptocurares.

La détermination de la séquence exacte des différents acides aminés dans chacune de ces toxines permettra de définir la nature et la position des acides aminés essentiels à l'activité biologique et peut-être d'expliquer la similitude entre des toxines provenant d'espèces ophidiennes très différentes, similitude d'effets pharmacologiques et biologiques, mais aussi similitude mise en évidence par Boque de propriétés immunologiques.

RESUME

L'activité, les propriétés immunologiques et la constitution chimique de quatre fractions isolées de venins appartenant à des espèces ophidiennes différentes sont comparées.

A partir des venins de quelques serpents dont les effets neuromusculaires sont maintenant mieux connus, il est possible d'isoler et de purifier par chromatographie ou électrophorèse la ou les fractions actives. Ainsi plusieurs fractions ont été étudiées et regroupées en fonction de la nature de leur action.

Action paralysante

L'α-najatoxine, isolée du venin de *Naja nigricollis* (Elapidé africian) et les erabutoxines a et b isolées du venin de *Laticauda semifasciata* (Hydrophidé japonais) produisent après latence une paralysie lente et progressive difficilement réversible. Cette action périphérique est due à un blocage des récepteurs de la plaque motrice.

Action contracturante

La crotamine, isolée du venin de *Crotalus durissus terrificus*, var. *crotaminicus* (serpent à sonnette brésilien) produit sur la Souris ou le Rat un syndrome spasmodique typique, susceptible de se répéter spontanément mais présentant le phénomène de tachyphylaxie. Sur préparations neuromusculaires isolées ou *in situ*, on observe une contracture immédiate avec difficultés de relaxation. Sur le *rectus abdominis* de Grenouille, on observe une sensibilisation au potassium. La crotamine agit sur la fibre musculaire en modifiant la perméabilité ou l'équilibre ionique.

References

Boquet, P., Y. Izard, J. Meaume et M. Jouannet 1966 'Etude de deux antigènes toxiques du venin de *Naja nigricollis*.' *Compt. Rend. Acad. Sci.*, **262**: 1134–1137.

Gonçalves, J. M. 1956 'Purification and properties of crotamine.' *In: Venoms,* Buckley, E. E. et N. Porges (eds.) pp. 261–274. A.A.A.S., Washington D.C.

Gonçalves, J. M. et J. R. Giglio 1964 'Amino-acid composition and terminal group analysis of crotamine.' *Proc. Sixth Int. Cong. Biochem.*, N.Y., **2**: 170.

Karlsson, E., D. L. Eaker et J. Porath 1966 'Purification of a neurotoxin from the venom of *Naja nigricollis*.' *Biochim. Biophys. Acta*, **127**: 505–520.

Tamiya, N. et H. Arai 1966 'Studies on sea snake venoms.' *Biochem. J.*, **99**: 624.

Tamiya, N., H. Arai et S. Sato 1967 'Studies on sea snakes venoms: crystallisation of erabutoxin "a" and "b" from *Laticauda semifasciata* venom and of Laticotoxin "a" from *Laticauda laticaudata* venom.' In: *Animal Toxins.* Russell, F. E. and P. R. Saunders (eds.), pp. 249–258. Pergamon Press, Oxford.

EFFECTS OF ß - BUNGAROTOXIN ON SYNAPTIC VESICLES

I-LI CHEN and C. Y. LEE

*Department of Anatomy and Pharmacological Institute, College of Medicine,
National Taiwan University, Taipei, Republic of China*

TWO KINDS of neurotoxins, called α- and β-bungarotoxin have been isolated from the venom of *Bungarus multicinctus* (banded krait) by means of zone electrophoresis on starch. α-Bungarotoxin produces a 'non-depolarising' type of neuromuscular block by acting on the postsynaptic membrane of the motor endplate, whereas β-bungarotoxin acts presynaptically, depressing acetylcholine release from the motor nerve endings and leaving the sensitivity of the endplate to acetylcholine unaffected (Chang and Lee, 1963). Subsequent studies have revealed that β-bungarotoxin causes complete disappearance of miniature endplate potentials (MEPPs) after a period of initial increase in the frequency of MEPPs (Lee and Chang, 1966).

The MEPPs are supposed to be due to spontaneous quantal release of acetylcholine from the axon terminals in the motor endplate (Fatt and Katz, 1952; Del Castillo and Katz, 1956). The presence of synaptic vesicles in the axon terminals has been postulated to link with the quantal packets of acetylcholine release (Katz, 1959; De Robertis, 1964).

The present work was started in the hope of obtaining any correlating morphological changes in the motor endplate with the observed electrophysiological effects of β-bungarotoxin.

MATERIALS AND METHODS

The bungarotoxins (α and β) were isolated from the venom of *Bungarus multicinctus* by column chromatography on CM-Sephadex (C-50) and further purified by rechromatography on CM-cellulose column. Both bungarotoxins have been shown to be free from any known enzyme activities, such as phospholipase A, acetylcholinesterase, diphosphopyridine nucleotidase (NADase), or phosphomonoesterase, which are present in the crude venom (Lee *et al.*, In preparation).

Sixteen adult albino mice (NIH strain) were injected intraperitoneally with 0.04–0.06 μg/g of β-bungarotoxin and sacrificed at 30 min, 1–1.5 hrs, and 2–4 hrs after envenomation. Four mice were injected with 0.4 μg/g of α-bungarotoxin and sacrificed immediately before death. Some other mice served as saline-injected controls. All mice were perfused with 3% glutaraldehyde in 0.1 M phosphate buffer (pH, 7.4) through the left ventricle. After perfusion the endplate zone of the diaphragm was cut into small pieces and further fixed with 3% glutaraldehyde followed by osmication. The tissues were then dehydrated and embedded in Epon. Thin sections were stained with lead citrate and examined with a Hitachi HU ll electron microscope.

RESULTS

In mice the fine structure of diaphragmatic endplatés is the same as that of intercostal ones (Zacks, 1964). The axon terminal of motor fibers fits into a small invagination in the surface of the muscle fiber. From the primary synaptic cleft numerous secondary clefts are derived. The normal axon terminal (Figure 1) is filled with numerous synaptic vesicles, a few elongated mitochondria and occasional bundles of fine neurofilaments. One or two profiles of small invaginations in the axolemma, which have been suggested as the opening of synaptic vesicles into the primary synaptic cleft (De Robertis, 1959), are encountered in some sections of axon terminals.

In accordance with the results described by Zacks (1964) using cobra (*Naja haje*) venom, neither decrease in the number of synaptic vesicles nor alteration in the ultrastructure of the endplates was observed with α-bungarotoxin, which is known to have a similar mode of action as cobra neurotoxin (Lee and Chang, 1966).

Following β-bungarotoxin administration some definite changes were observed in the axon terminals in the endplates. In general, 30 min after envenomation, increased profiles of opened synaptic vesicles at the axolemma were observed in the nerve terminal. However, the structure and number of

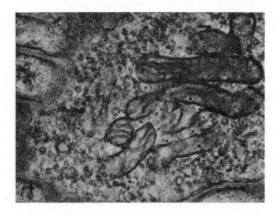

FIGURE 1.   Motor endplate of a control mouse. The axon terminal is filled with numerous synaptic vesicles and a few elongated mitochondria 33,000 x

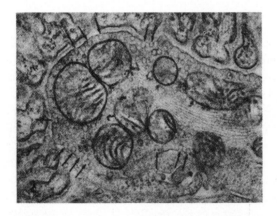

FIGURE 2.   Motor endplate of the mouse sacrificed one hour after β-bungarotoxin injection. A marked decrease in number of synaptic vesicles in the axon terminal and numerous profiles of opened synaptic vesicles (arrows) at the axolemma are seen. The axoplasmic mitochondria appear to be swollen and spheroid in shape 33,000 x

synaptic vesicles and mitochondria in the axon terminals appeared to be unchanged. During 1 to 1.5 hrs after injection a considerable decrease in the number of synaptic vesicles was found, accompanied by an increase in profiles of opened synaptic vesicles at the axolemma (Figure 2). Early in this

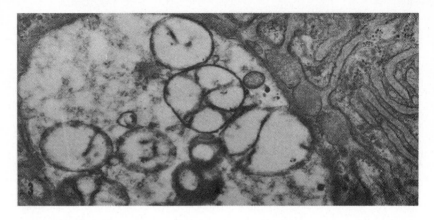

FIGURE 3.   Motor endplate of the mouse sacrificed two hours after β-bungarotoxin injection. The synaptic vesicles in the axon terminal have almost completely disappeared and the axonal mitochondria are swollen and vacuolated. The mitochondria in the muscle fiber appear to be morphologically normal 33,000 x

stage the mitochondria in the axon terminals began to swell and vacuolization of the mitochondria took place late in this stage. Two to 4 hrs after injection the synaptic vesicles in the axon terminals disappeared almost completely and profiles of opened vesicles were encountered only occasionally. Vacuolization of the mitochondria in the axon terminals became prominent and fusion of smaller vacuoles into larger ones in the mitochondria occurred. As a result, the terminal axons were filled with swollen and vacuolated mitochondria, with a few vesicles which were usually larger in diameter than the normal ones, and a fine granular or flocculent matrix (Figure 3). Throughout all the phases following β-bungarotoxin injection the fine structure of muscle fibers, fibrocytes, endothelial cells and myelinated axons in the muscle appeared to be normal.

DISCUSSION

Attempts have been made to deplete synaptic vesicles in the nerve endings by various means. De Robertis (1964) claimed that high frequency electrical stimulation of the splanchnic nerve caused a depletion of synaptic vesicles within the cholinergic nerve endings of the adrenal medulla. However, Birks *et al.* (1960) were unsuccessful in obtaining similar findings from muscles which had been subjected to even drastic synaptic stimulation (i.e., exposure to high potassium concentration and hypertonic media). Experiments with botulinum toxin, which is known to prevent the release of acetylcholine from the cholinergic nerve endings, also revealed no abnormalities in the ultra-structure of motor endplates (Thesleff, 1960; Zacks *et al.*, 1962). Moderate swelling and vacuolization of axoplasmic mitochondria found in some end-plates poisoned with botulinum toxin were interpreted as being due to arti-facts resulting from fixation and embedding (Zacks *et al.*, 1962). The marked increase in profiles of opened synaptic vesicles at the axolemma, accompanied with a considerable depletion of synaptic vesicles within the axon terminals observed in this study suggests that the opened synaptic vesicles at the axolemma represent a releasing rather than an absorbing (Birks *et al.*, 1960) process in the axon terminals. These morphological findings, coupled with the pharmacological data showing that β-bungarotoxin markedly increases the frequency of MEPPs in the early stage of intoxication (Lee and Chang, 1966), provide a strong support to the hypothesis that acetylcholine is stored in synaptic vesicles and released from the axon terminals in quantal packets (Katz, 1959; De Robertis, 1964). This view is further strengthened by the findings that the synaptic vesicles in the axon terminals disappear almost completely during the later stage of intoxication, when the release of acetyl-choline from the motor nerve endings is severely depressed (Chang and Lee, 1963) and the MEPPs disappear almost completely (Lee and Chang, 1966).

The exact mechanism by which β-bungarotoxin exerts its effect on the motor nerve endings is not well understood. The swelling and vacuolization of the axoplasmic mitochondria observed in our material do not seem to be merely due to fixation and embedding artifacts as proposed for the findings obtained with botulinum toxin (Zacks *et al.*, 1962), since progressive swelling and vacuolization of axonal mitochondria were consistently observed after administration of β-bungarotoxin. These changes are not due to phospholi-pase A, a mitochondrial poison contained in the crude venoms, since β-bungarotoxin is free from such enzyme activity. It is also unlikely that β-bungarotoxin directly interferes with acetylcholine synthesis since it does not inhibit acetylation of choline by brain extracts in the presence of ATP (Lee, unpublished observation). However, it is possible that β-bungarotoxin selec-tively affects the membrane of the motor nerve endings, accelerating the release of vesicle content on one hand and exerting some metabolic effects on the axonal mitochondria on the other, consequently shutting off the energy supply for the resynthesis of acetylcholine in the nerve terminals (De Robertis, 1964). As a result, neuromuscular blockade takes place due to exhaustion of acetylcholine stores in the motor nerve endings.

SUMMARY

β-Bungarotoxin, isolated from *Bungarus multicinctus* venom, induced an increase in the profiles of opened synaptic vesicles at the axolemma, accompanied by a decrease in number of synaptic vesicles and subsequently, almost complete depletion of the vesicles in the axon terminal of motor endplates. The toxin also caused progressive swelling and vacuolization of the mitochondria in the motor nerve endings.

References

Birks, R., H. E. Huxley and B. Katz 1960 'The fine structure of the neuromuscular junction of the frog.' *J. Physiol.*, (London), **150**: 134–144.

Chang, C. C. and C. Y. Lee 1963 'Isolation of neurotoxins from the venom of *Bungarus multicinctus* and their modes of neuromuscular blocking action.' *Arch. Int. Pharmacodyn.*, **144** : 241–257.

De Robertis, E. 1959 'Submicroscopic morphology of the synapse.' *Int. Rev. Cytol.*, **8**: 61–96.

De Robertis, E. 1964 '*Histophysiology of Synapses and Neurosecretions.*' Pergamon Press, Oxford.

Del Castillo, J. and B. Katz 1956 'Biophysical aspects of neuromuscular transmission.' *Progr. Biophys.*, **6** : 121–170.

Fatt, P. and B. Katz 1952 'Spontaneous subthreshold activity at motor nerve endings.' *J. Physiol.*, (London), **117**: 109–128.

Katz, B. 1959 'Mechanisms of synaptic transmission.' *Rev. Mod. Phys.*, **31**: 524–531.

Lee, C. Y. and C. C. Chang 1966 'Modes of actions of purified toxins from elapid venoms on neuromuscular transmission.' *Mem. Inst. Butantan, Simp. Internac.*, **33**: 555–572.

Lee, C. Y., S. L. Chang and S. T. Kau 'Chromatographic separation of the venom of *Bungarus multicinctus* on CM-Sephadex and CM-cellulose columns.' In preparation.

Thesleff, S. 1960 'Supersensitivity of skeletal muscle produced by botulinum toxin.' *J. Physiol.*, (London), **161**: 598–607.

Zacks, S. I. 1964 '*The Motor Endplate.*' W. B. Saunders Co., Philadelphia.

Zacks, S. I., J. F. Metzger, J. F. Smith and J. M. Blumber 1962 'Localization of ferritin-labelled botulinus.toxin in the neuromuscular junction of the mouse.' *J. Neuropathol. Exptl. Neur.*, **21**: 610–633.

THE ACTION OF DIRECT LYTIC AGENTS FROM ANIMAL VENOMS ON CELLS AND ISOLATED CELL FRACTIONS

E. KAISER, R. KRAMAR and R. LAMBRECHTER

*Department of Medical Chemistry, School of Medicine,
University of Vienna, Vienna, Austria*

INTRODUCTION

IT HAS BEEN DEMONSTRATED that lysis of washed erythrocytes by cobra venom is produced by the synergistic action of two venom components: a basic polypeptide which is slightly hemolytic by itself, named direct lytic factor (DLF), and the venom phospholipase A which is not hemolytic when applied alone (Condrea *et al.*, 1964a, 1964b, 1965; Kirschmann *et al.*, 1964). Melittin, another direct hemolytic principle has been isolated from bee venom (Habermann and Reiz, 1965; Kreil, 1965; Habermann, 1968). Most of the cytolytic bacterial toxins damage cells directly without an enzyme (Bernheimer, 1968).

In order to obtain more information on the mechanism of action of direct lytic agents we investigated whether direct hemolytic agents have a cytotoxic action on other types of cells and on isolated cell fractions. In addition, some experiments on the possible receptor compound for DLF on the red cell surface were performed.

Preparations of DLF and phospholipase A were obtained from cobra venom (*Naja naja*) by established methods (Condrea *et al.*, 1964a; Slotta and Vick, 1969), and some preparations of DLF were kindly supplied by Professor Slotta.

EFFECTS ON RABBIT PLATELETS IN VITRO (CF. KAISER *ET AL.*, (1970a)

We have investigated in some detail the effect of DLF on rabbit platelets *in vitro* using a method developed by Bernheimer and Schwartz (1965). The results of these experiments are illustrated in Table 1.

TABLE 1   Effects of direct lytic factor on platelets

Treatment of platelets	Per cent decrease in O.D.	Per cent release of	
		proteins	nucleic acids
—	2–4	3–5	3–6
5 cycles of freezing and thawing	—	100	100
cobra venom (1 mg/ml)	63	52	66
DLF (100 μg/ml)	25	29	34
phospholipase A (100 μg/ml)	6	8	10
DLF + phospholipase A	84	59	76

Methods (cf. Bernheimer and Schwartz, 1965)
Platelets: 9 parts rabbit blood + 1 part Na citrate (3.8%), 15 min/400 g; supernatant 10 min/20,000 g; suspension in phosphate buffered saline, pH 7.
Turbidity measurements: Beckman recording spectrophotometer at 520 nm, 37°, 20 min.
Proteins, nucleic acids: centrifugation at 20,000 g, 15 min, 4°, UV-absorption measurements at 260 and 280 nm.

EFFECTS ON RAT PERITONEAL MAST CELLS (CF. KAISER *ET AL.*, 1970b)

The synergistic action of DLF and phospholipase A is not restricted to red cells and platelets. Table 2 shows the results obtained with rat peritoneal mast cells (Rothschild, 1965; Kaiser *et al.*, 1970b).

EFFECTS ON FIBROBLASTS AND TUMOR CELLS

Dr Springer in our laboratory has demonstrated that several direct lytic agents have a cytotoxic activity against human fibroblasts in tissue culture and against Ehrlich's ascites cells of the mouse.

TABLE 2   Effects of direct lytic factor on rat peritoneal mast cells

Treatment of mast cells	Per cent histamine release
–	8
Compound 48/80 (5 μg/ml)	100
cobra venom (100 μg/ml)	68
DLF (10 μg/ml)	29
phospholipase A (100 μg/ml)	6
DLF + phospholipase A	82

Methods (cf. Rothschild, 1965)
Mast cells: i.p. injection of Tyrose solution (+ 1 mg serum albumin/ml); several washings of peritoneal cell suspension (cf. Rothschild, 1965)
Incubation period: 10 min at 37°.
Histamine: fluorometric method (Shohre, *et al.*, 1959)

EFFECTS ON RAT LIVER LYSOSOMES (CF. KRAMAR *ET AL.*, 1970)

Several agents which cause injury to erythrocytes are also capable of releasing hydrolytic enzymes from lysosomes (Weissmann and Thomas, 1962; Kramar *et al.*, 1970). Our experiments have shown a synergistic effect of DLF and phospholipase A on lysosomes from rat liver (Kramar *et al.*, 1970). The results of these experiments are illustrated in Table 3.

POSSIBLE RECEPTOR FOR DLF IN THE RED CELL MEMBRANE

The mechanism of action of DLF on erythrocytes is not known, neither is the receptor in the red cell membrane. Several attempts have been made to elucidate the action of direct lytic agents.

Red cell sensitivity to DLF is in good agreement with red cell permeability for certain agents and with their phospholipid content (Condrea *et al.*, 1964b). It is well known that the lytic action of several bacterial toxins is inhibited by cholesterol, phospholipids or sphingomyelin in small concentrations (cf. Bernheimer, 1968). From these results it has been concluded that these inhibitors might be the specific receptors for the toxins.

We have performed inactivation experiments with cobra venom DLF using a method developed by Howard *et al.* (1953). Solutions of phosphatidylcholine in ligroin were exposed to a solution of DLF in buffered saline in an apparatus devised by the authors. In control experiments ligroin alone was

TABLE 3   Effects of direct lytic factor on lysosomes from rat liver

Treatment of lysosomes	Per cent release of		
	β-glucuronidase	acid phosphatase	cathepsin
Triton X-100 (1 mg/ml)	100	100	100
phospholipase A (100 μg/ml)	28	30	0
DLF (400 μg/ml)	50	14	0
phospholipase A + DLF	91	69	260

Methods:
The lysosomes contained in the large granular fraction from rat liver were prepared according to Weissmann and Thomas (1962). Particles were incubated at 37° for 15 minutes. After centrifugation (20 min, 37.000 g/4°) acid phosphatase (Gutman and Gutman, 1940), cathepsin (Anson, 1937) and β-glucuronidase (Gianetto and de Duve, 1955) were determined in the supernatant. Enzymatic activity solubilized from lysosomes by Triton X-100 was taken as 100% (Wittiaux and de Duve, 1956).

TABLE 4   Effects of treatment of DLF with phosphatidylcholine on hemolytic activity

	Erythrocytes from		
	guinea pig	man	sheep
Content of phosphatidylcholine (per cent of total P-lipids) (Nelson 1967)	41.1	27.2	0
DLF (hemolysis, per cent)	36	7	1
DLF treated with phosphatidylcholine (hemolysis, per cent)	28	6	2

Methods
Treatment of DLF: 2 mg/ml DLF in 0.15 M NaCl, pH 7.4 + solution of phosphatidylcholine in ligroin according to Howard *et al.* (1953).
Hemolysis: 1 ml packed cells + 0.5 ml DLF solution (2 hrs/37°); determination of hemoglobin released, calculated in per cent of total hemoglobin present (cf. Condrea *et al.*, 1964b).

TABLE 5   Action of DLF and phospholipase A on neuraminidase treated human erythrocytes

	Per cent hemolysis (2 hrs/37°)	
	untreated	neuraminidase treated
—	2.0	2.2
DLF	3.1	7.2
phospholipase A	1.8	20.2
phospholipase A + DLF	69.7	59.8

Methods
Treatment of red cells: RDE (Behring Werke/Marburg) in 0.145 M NaCl + 0.005 M calcium chloride + erythrocytes, 1 hr/37°. Several washings.
Hemolysis: 1 ml packed cells + 0.5 ml DLF (1.5 mg/ml) or 0.5 ml phospholipase A (1.5 mg/ml), 2 hrs at 37°. Determination of hemoglobin released, calculated in per cent of total hemoglobin present.

passed through the DLF solution. The results of these experiments are illustrated in Table 4. The results demonstrate that a correlation exists between phosphatidylcholine content of red cells from various animal species (Nelson, 1967) and its susceptibility to DLF (cf. Condrea *et al.*, 1969b). However, treatment of DLF with phosphatidylcholine does not reduce its hemolytic activity. Therefore it seems unlikely that this compound is involved in the lytic action of DLF.

Since DLF is a basic polypeptide, the negative surface charge of the red cell might be responsible for the binding of DLF to the erythrocyte. Condrea *et al.* (1964b) have already discussed the role of the negative charge of red cells in determining the adsorption of DLF to erythrocytes. Although it was shown that there is no correlation between the negative charge of red cells from various animal species and the sensitivity to DLF we have taken up this question again. The negative surface charge of red cells, mostly due to the neuraminic acid, is greatly reduced by treatment with neuraminidase (Eylar *et al.*, 1962; Seaman and Uhlenbruck, 1963; Uhlenbruck *et al.*, 1967; Uhlenbruck and Pardoe, 1968). We have investigated the action of DLF and phospholipase A on neuraminidase treated red cells and the results of this experiment are shown in Table 5.

Neuraminidase treated red cells became sensitive to phospholipase A, which is inactive against untreated cells. It might be possible that the basic polypeptide DLF is bound to the anionic groups of neuraminic acid on the red cell surface. Binding of DLF to the cell membrane might induce a new arrangement in the surface components unmasking substrates susceptible to phospholipase A. Since other basic substances such as protamine (Becker, 1961) or polylysin which can produce hemolysis, are not 'activators' for phospholipase A at the red cell membrane (Condrea et al., 1964a) it may be assumed that the effect of DLF on the cell membrane is highly specific. This hypothetic mechanism is further supported by our observation that following neuraminidase treatment, red cells become sensitive to the acidic protein phospholipase A.

The synergistic action of DLF and phospholipase A on other types of membranes might be explained by a similar mechanism. It is known that the membranes of platelets (Born, 1968), tumor cells (Wallach and de Perez Esandi, 1964) and lysosomes (Sawant et al., 1964) are negatively charged mostly because of their content of neuraminic acid.

SUMMARY

The synergistic action of the direct lytic factor (DLF) and phospholipase A from cobra venom is not restricted to red cells. A similar synergism is found using platelets, mast cells, tumor cells and isolated cell fractions (lysosomes from rat liver). Neuraminidase treated red cells become sensitive to phospholipase A which is inactive against untreated cells. It is suggested that the basic polypeptide DLF is bound to the anionic groups of neuraminic acid on the red cell surface. Binding of DLF to the cell surface might induce a new arrangement of the surface components unmasking susceptible substrates to phospholipase A. Since other basic substances (protamine, polylysin) are not 'activators' for phospholipase A at the red cell membrane it is assumed that the effect of DLF on the cell membrane is highly specific.

References

Anson, M. L. 1937 'Estimation of cathespsin with hemoglobin and the partial purification of cathepsin.' *J. Gen. Physiol.*, **20**: 565.

Becker, F. F. 1961 'Studies on the hemolytic properties of protamine.' *J. Gen. Physiol.*, **44**:433.

Bernheimer, A. W. 1968 'Cytolytic toxins of bacterial origin.' *Science*, **159**: 847.

Bernheimer, A. W. and L. L. Schwartz 1965 'Effects of staphylococcal and other bacterial toxins on platelets in vitro.' *J. Pathol. Bacteriol.*, **89**: 209.

Born, V. R. 1968 'The platelet membrane and its function.' *In*: Deutsch, E., E. Gerlach and K. Moser (eds.), *Metabolism and Membrane Permeability of Erythrocytes and Thrombocytes.* p. 294. G. Thieme, Stuttgart.

Condrea, E., A. de Vries and J. Mager 1964a 'Hemolysis and splitting of human erythrocyte phospholipids by snake venom.' *Biochim. Biophys. Acta*, **84**: 60.

Condrea, E., I. Kendzersky and A. de Vries 1965 'Binding of Ringhals venom direct hemolytic factor to erythrocytes and osmotic ghosts of various animal species.' *Experientia*, **21**: 461.

Condrea, E., Z. Mammon, S. Aloof and A. de Vries 1964b 'Susceptibility of erythrocytes of various animal species to the hemolytic and phospholipid splitting of snake venoms.' *Biochim. Biophys. Acta*, **84**: 365.

Eylar, E. H., M. A. Madoff, O. V. Brody and J. L. Oncley 1962 'The contribution of sialic acid to the surface charge of the erythrocyte.' *J. Biol. Chem.*, **237**: 1992.

Habermann, E. 1968 'Biochemie, Pharmakologie und Toxikologie der Inhaltsstoffe von Hymenopterengiften.' *Ergebn. Physiologie*, **60**: 220.

Gianetto, R. and C. de Duve 1955 'Tissue fractionation studies. 4. Comparative study of the binding of acid phosphatase, β-glucuronidase and cathepsin by rat-liver particles.' *Biochem. J.*, **59**: 433.

Gutman, E. B. and A. B. Gutman 1940 'Estimation of "acid" phosphatase activity of blood serum.' *J. Biol. Chem.*, **136**: 201.

Habermann, E. and K. G. Reiz 1965 'Zur Biochemie der Bienengiftpeptide Melittin und Apamin.' *Biochem. Z.*, **343**: 192.

Howard, J. G., K. R. Wallace and G. P. Wright 1953 'The inhibitory effects of cholesterol and related sterols on hemolysis by streptolysin O.' *Brit. J. Exptl. Pathol.*, **34**: 174.

Kaiser, E., R. Kramar and F. Mayer 1970a 'Effects of cobra venom on rabbit platelets *in vitro*.' (In preparation.)

Kaiser, E., R. Kramar and M. M. Müller 1970b 'Histamine release from mast cells by cobra venom.' (In preparation.)

Kirschmann, C., E. Condrea, N. Moav, S. Aloof and A. de Vries 1964 'Action of snake venom on human platelet phospholipids.' *Arch. Int. Pharmacodyn. Therap.*, **150**: 372.

Kramar, R., R. Lambrechter and E. Kaiser 1970 'The release of acid hydrolases from lysosomes by animal venoms.' Toxicon **9**: 125.

Kreil, G. 1965 'Isolation and characterization of melittin, the principal toxin of bee venom.' *Monatsh. Chem.*, **96**: 2061.

Nelson, G. J. 1967 'Lipid composition of erythrocytes in various mammalian species.' *Biochim. Biophys. Acta*, **144**: 221.

Rothschild, A. M. 1965 'Histamine release by bee venom phospholipase A and melittin in the rat.' *Brit. J. Pharmacol.*, **25**: 59.

Sawant, P. L., I. D. Desai and A. L. Tappel 1964 'Factors affecting the lysosomal membrane and availability of enzymes.' *Arch. Biochem. Biophys.*, 105: 247.

Seaman, G. V. F. and G. Uhlenbruck 1963 'The surface structure of erythrocytes from some animal sources.' *Arch. Biochem. Biophys.*, 100: 493.

Shohre, P. A., A. Burkhalter and V. H. Cohn Jr 1959 'A method for the fluorometric assay of histamine in tissues.' *J. Pharmacol.*, 127: 182.

Slotta, K. H. and J. A. Vick 1969 'Identification of the direct lytic factor from cobra venom as cardiotoxin.' *Toxicon.* 6: 167.

Uhlenbruck, G. und C. J. Pardoe 1968 'Die Struktur der Erythrozytenoberfläche.' *In*: Deutsch, E., E. Gerlach and K. Moser (eds.), *Metabolism and Membrane permeability of Erythrocytes and Thrombocytes*. p. 342. G. Thieme, Stuttgart.

Uhlenbruck, G., G. Wintzer und R. Wersdörder 1967 'Studien über den Aufbau der Zellmembran, insbesondere derjenigen des roten Blutkörperchens.' *Z. Klin. Chem. Klin. Biochem.*, 5: 281.

Wallach, D. F. H. and M. V. de Perez Esandi 1964 'Sialic acid and the electrophoretic mobility of three tumor cell types.' *Biochim. Biophys. Acta*, 83: 363.

Wattiaux, R. and C. de Duve 1956 'Tissue fractionation studies. 7. Release of bound hydrolases by means of Triton X-100.' *Biochem. J.*, 63: 606.

Weissmann, G. and L. Thomas 1962 'Studies on lysosomes. I. The effects of endotoxin, endotoxin tolerance and cortisone on release of acid hydrolases from a granular fractions of rabbit liver.' *J. Exptl.*, 116: 433.

THE EFFECT OF SNAKE AND BEE VENOMS ON CARDIOVASCULAR HEMODYNAMICS AND FUNCTION

S. J. PHILLIPS, M.D.*

Division of Surgery, Walter Reed Army Institute of Research,
Walter Reed Army Medical Center, Washington, D.C., U.S.A.

THE PRESENT STUDY was undertaken to describe the early sequential hemodynamic changes in an animal model in which doses of snake and bee venoms were administered, intravenously or by direct bite, in anesthetized dogs on assisted ventilation.

MATERIALS AND METHODS

Experimental protocol

Fourteen venoms were administered to twenty-eight anesthetized (sodium pentobarbital) mongrel dogs weighing between 10–12 kgs. Lyophilized doses of snake and bee venoms were injected intravenously in the experimental model. Snake venoms representative of Elapidae, Crotalidae, Viperidae and Hydrophidae families and venoms obtained from bees in the United States and Russia were used.

Table 1 lists the venoms and doses used.

All experiments were conducted acutely. Endotracheal intubation and assisted ventilation with a model 607 Harvard pump was initiated. Through a left fourth or fifth interspace thoracotomy the pericardium was opened and large bore polyethylene catheters (Clay-Adams PE 205) were inserted into the main pulmonary artery and right and left atria. A calibrated Biotronex Labor-

*Department of Surgery, Sinai Hospital, Detroit, Michigan

TABLE 1

Venom	Dose
Bee Venoms	
Russian	10.0 mg/kg
American phospholipase A	3.0 mg/kg
Active surfactant	0.8 mg/kg
Melittin	5.0 mg/kg
Snake Venoms	
Crotalidae	
Crotalus h. horridus	Bite (approx. 3 mg/kg)
Agkistrodon piscivorus	10.0 mg/kg
Lachesis mutus	1.0 mg/kg
Crotalus adamanteus	10.0 mg/kg
Viperidae	
Bitis gabonica	6 mg/kg
Vipera aspis	1.8 mg/kg
Elapidae	
Ophiophagus hannah	Bite (approx. 1.5 mg/kg)
Naja naje	1.5 mg/kg
Dendroaspis angusticeps	1.5 mg/kg
Hydrophidae	
Laticauda semifasciata	1.0 mg/kg

atory flow probe was placed around the main pulmonary artery. Another catheter was introduced into the right femoral artery. The electrocardiogram was recorded via bilateral subcutaneous chest needle electrodes.

Methods of hemodynamic measurement

Continuous recordings of all measured parameters and assisted ventilation were used throughout all experiments.

Duplicate experiments were performed for each venom studied.

Pulmonary arterial flow was measured with a Biotronex Laboratory 310 sine wave electromagnetic flow meter. The right and left atrial catheters were connected to 268B Sanborn pressure transducers and the pulmonary and femoral arterial catheters were connected to 267AC Sanborn pressure transducers.

Electrocardiogram, heart rate, pulmonary arterial flow, pulmonary arterial pressure, right and left atrial pressures and femoral arterial pressure were simultaneously measured and recorded on an eight channel direct writing Hewlett-Packard recorder.

Pulmonary vascular resistance (PVR) and systemic vascular resistance (SVR) were measured in $\dfrac{\text{Dyne-second}}{\text{centimeter}}$ and were derived using the following formulae:

$$PVR = \frac{mPAP\text{-}LAP}{CO} \times 7{,}992;$$

$$SVR = \frac{mAP\text{-}RAP}{CO} \times 7{,}992$$

where mPAP is mean pulmonary arterial pressure, LAP is left atrial pressure; mAP is mean arterial pressure, RAP is right atrial pressure; both arterial and atrial pressures are expressed in mm Hg. Left (LVSW) and right ventricular stroke work (RVSW) were *measured in gram-meters and* were calculated according to the formulae:

$$LVSW = \frac{SV \times mAP \times 13.5}{1{,}000}$$

$$RVSW = \frac{SV \times mPAP \times 13.5}{1{,}000}$$

Average stroke volume (SV) was determined by dividing cardiac output by the heart rate. Cardiac output was calculated from the pulmonary arterial flow curve. All calculations were solved by an Olivetti-Underwood 101 electronic computer programmed for this purpose.

In conducting the research described in this report, the investigators adhered to the 'Guide for Laboratory Animal Facilities and Care,' as promulgated by the Committee on Revision of the Guide for Laboratory Animal Facilities and Care of the Institute of Laboratory Animal Resources, National Academy of Sciences—National Research Council.

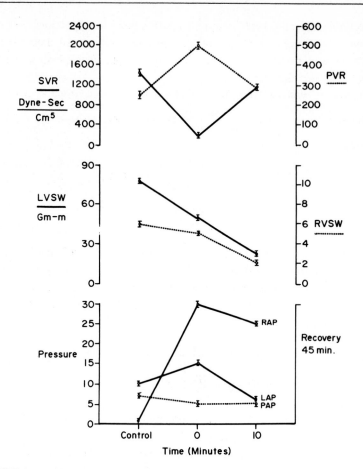

FIGURE 1.   Effects of Russian bee venom

Abbreviations

PVR   = Pulmonary vascular resistance
SVR   = Systemic vascular resistance
PVR and SVR are measured in Dyne-seconds
                              centimeter[5]
LVSW   = Left ventricular stroke work
RVSW   = Right ventricular stroke work
LVSW and RVSW are measured in Grams-Meter
RAP   = Right atrial pressure
LAP   = Left atrial pressure
PAP   = Pulmonary artery pressure
RAP, LAP, PAP, blood pressure are measured in millimeters of Mercury (mm Hg)

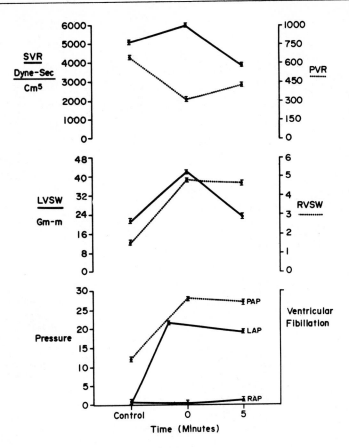

FIGURE 2. Effects of phospholipase A. Abbreviations as in Figure 1

RESULTS AND DISCUSSION

Bee venoms

Figures 1 through 4 summarize the results of intravenous injections of Russian bee venom and mellitin, phospholipase A and the active surfactant fractions of the American bee venom.

The Russian bee venom (Figure 1) caused an initial precipitous fall in the systemic vascular resistance with a concomitant rise in the pulmonary vascular resistance with the return of both to the baseline within 10 minutes.

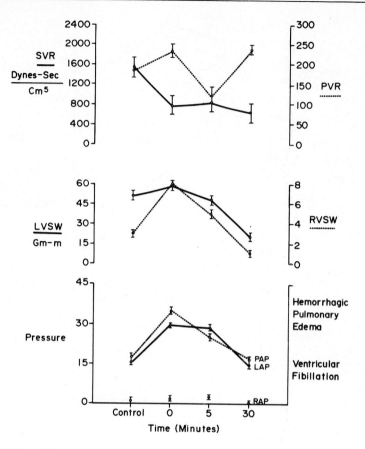

FIGURE 3.   Effects of active surfactant. Abbreviations as in Figure 1

A fall in the right and left ventricular stroke work with elevation of both right and left atrial pressures occurred indicating transient heart failure. Due to the decrease in systemic vascular resistance the resistive load on the left ventricle was decreased and left heart failure was not as evident as right heart failure (markedly elevated right atrial pressure). Hemodynamic recovery occurred in 45 minutes. Injection of phospholipase A (Figure 2) and active surfactant (Figure 3) caused ventricular fibrillation after 5 and 30 minutes respectively. With active surfactant acute pulmonary hypertension and profound hemorrhagic pulmonary edema occurred prior to death.

The melittin fraction (Figure 4) of American bee venom caused acute pulmonary hypertension and right ventricular failure within 15 minutes of administration and death due to cardiac failure after three hours.

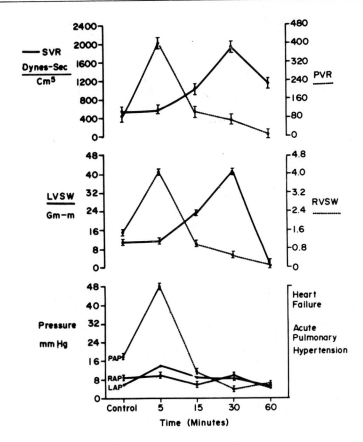

FIGURE 4.   Effects of mellitin. Abbreviations as in Figure 1

Snake venoms

Figures 5 through 8 summarize the effects of the venoms of the family Crotalidae: Water moccasin (*Agkistrodon piscivorus*)—Figure 5, Eastern Diamond Back (*Crotalus adamanteus*)—Figure 6, Bushmaster (*Lachesis muta*)—Figure 7, and Timber Rattlesnake (*Crotalus h. horridus*)—Figure 8; all venoms caused similar hemodynamic responses. Decreases in ventricular stroke work, elevation of the systemic and pulmonary vascular resistances, and biventricular cardiac failure occurred in all. Ventricular fibrillation occurred within 30 minutes with all but the Timber Rattlesnake. In this latter

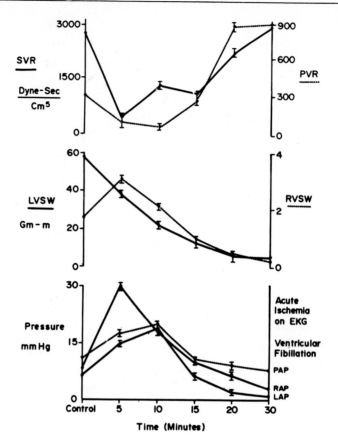

FIGURE 5.   Effects of *Agkistrodon piscivorus* venom. Abbreviations as in Figure 1

case, envenomation occurred by direct bite and the dose of venom was unknown. This study indicates that the primary toxicity of *Crotalus* venom is myocardial rather than pulmonary (Russell *et al.*, 1962; Halmagyl *et al.*, 1965; Russell, 1967).

Venoms of the Gaboon Viper (*Bitis gabonica*) Figure 9 and the European Asp (*Vipera aspis*) Figure 10 of the Viperidae family caused death within 60

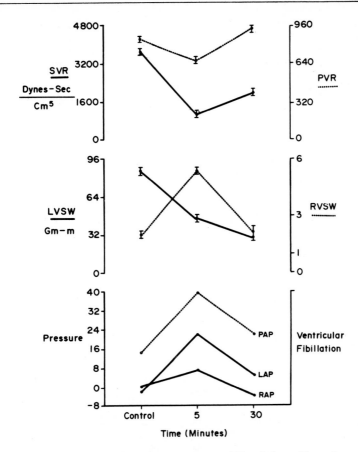

FIGURE 6.   Effects of *Crotalus adamanteus* venom. Abbreviations—Figure 1

minutes. Both venoms caused elevations of the systemic and pulmonary vascular resistances with concomitant fall in cardiac stroke work. Envenomation by the European Asp caused hemorrhagic pulmonary edema and cardiac standstill; whereas Gaboon viper venom caused no gross pulmonary manifestations but created ventricular fibrillation at 60 minutes.

Venoms representative of the families Elapidae (Figures 11 through 13)

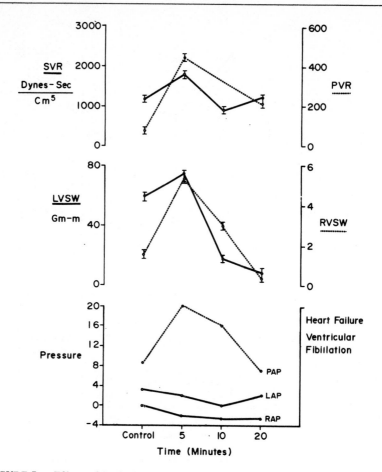

FIGURE 7.   Effects of *Lachesis muta* venom. Abbreviations—Figure 1

caused initial cardiac failure as manifested by varying degrees of reduction in ventricular stroke work. Hemodynamic recovery occurred in all. These venoms have been shown to be primarily neurotoxic (Russell *et al.*, 1961; Vick *et al.*, 1964, 1965; Bicher *et al.*, 1965).

Sea Snake venom (*Laticauda semifasciata*), Figure 14, from the family Hydrophidae caused essentially no immediate hemodynamic changes other than an initial blood pressure fall. It has been shown that this venom acts primarily on the post-synaptic membrane and death is due to respiratory paralysis (Tamiya *et al.*, 1967).

Venoms are complex mixtures, some containing as many as 15 or 20

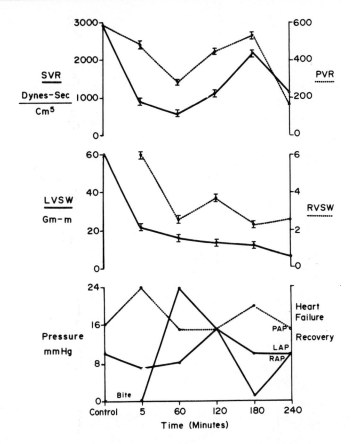

FIGURE 8.   Effects of *Crotalus horridus* venom. Abbreviations–Figure 1

specific biologically active components (Russell, 1967). Besides the individual components of venoms, the envenomated organism can produce and release autopharmacological substances which may not only complicate the poisoning but which may in themselves sometimes produce more serious consequences than the venom.

Though venoms have been studied extensively (Russell and Scharffenberg, 1964), their chemical composition and most of the specific physiopharmacological effects of these poisons and their fractions have not yet been determined.

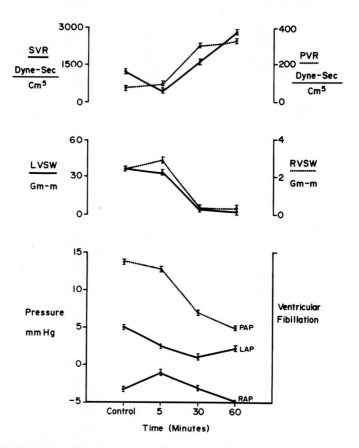

FIGURE 9.   Effects of *Bitis gabonica* venom. Abbreviations–Figure 1

The inadequate but widely accepted classification of venoms into 'neuro-toxins', 'hemotoxins', and 'cardiotoxins', led the author to design his study to eliminate as much as possible the 'neurotoxic' and 'hemotoxic' effects of venoms. Assisted ventilation was utilized to eliminate the secondary effects of anoxia (due to respiratory paralysis) on cardiovascular function. Acute, rather

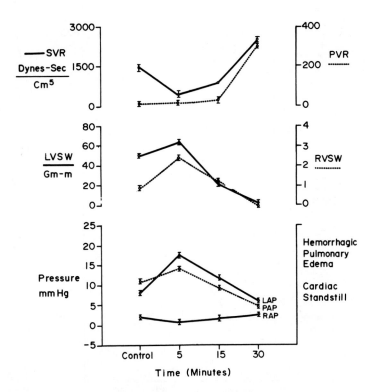

FIGURE 10.   Effects of *Vipera aspis* venom. Abbreviations—Figure 1

than chronic studies were performed to eliminate the delayed 'hemotoxic' and autopharmacological effects of these venoms.

Table 2 summarizes the cardiovascular and pulmonary effects of all venoms studied.

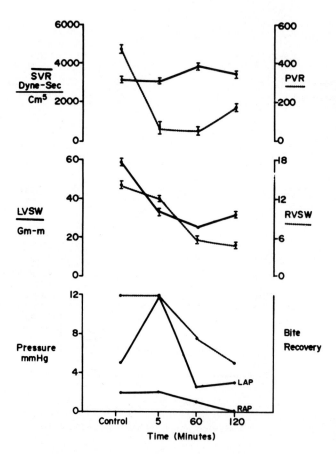

FIGURE 11.   Effects of *Ophiophagus hannah* venom. Abbreviations—Figure 1

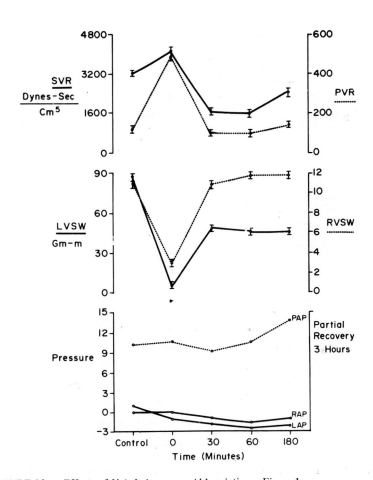

FIGURE 12.   Effects of *Naja haje* venom. Abbreviations—Figure 1

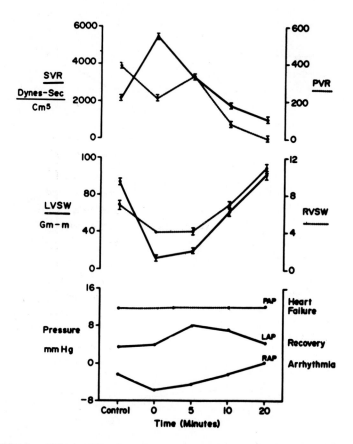

FIGURE 13.   Effects of *Dendroaspis angusticeps* venom. Abbreviations–Figure 1

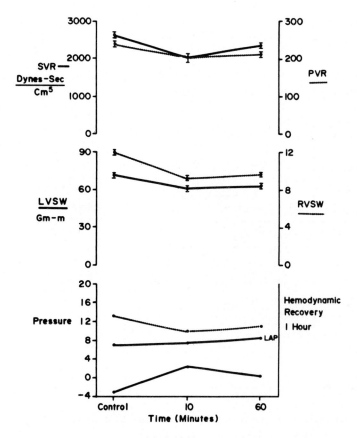

FIGURE 14.   Effects of *Laticauda semifasciata* venom. Abbreviations—Figure 1

TABLE 2   Summary of the immediate effects of venoms on cardiac and pulmonary function

	Cardiac	Pulmonary	Time to Death (Min)
Bee Venoms			
Russian	Transient*	None	Recovery
American phospholipase A	Profound*	Minimal	5
Active surfactant	Profound	Profound*	30
Mellitin	Profound	Profound*	180
Snake Venoms			
Crotalidae	Profound*	Moderate	30 (recovery from Timber Rattlesnake bite)
Viperidae	Profound	Profound (Asp)*	60
Elapidae	Mild*	None	Recovery
Hydrophidae	None	None	Recovery

*Denotes primary effect

SUMMARY

The cardiovascular effects of intravenous doses of snake and bee venoms were studied in open chest ventilated mongrel dogs.

The fractions of American bee venom caused acute pulmonary hypertension followed by cardiac failure indicating that their primary mode of action is on the pulmonary vascular circulation. The Russian bee venom, on the other hand seemed to have a direct toxic effect on the myocardium.

Representative venoms of the families Crotalidae and Elapidae had direct myocardial toxic effects while those of the Viperidae had their primary effects on both the pulmonary vascular bed and myocardium.

References

Bicher, H. I., C. Klibansky, J. Shiloah, S. Gitter and A. de Vries 1965 'Isolation of three different neurotoxins from Indian cobra venom and the relation of their action to phospholipase A.' *Biochem. Pharmacol.*, 14 : 1779.

Halmagyl, D. F. J., B. Starzecki and G. J. Horner 1965 'Mechanism and pharmacology of shock due to rattlesnake venom in sheep.' *J. Appl. Physiol.*, 20: 709–718.

Russell, F. E. 1967 'Pharmacology of animal venoms.' *Clin. Pharmacol. Therap.*, 8: 849–871.

Russell, F. E., F. W. Buess and J. Strassberg 1962 'Cardiovascular response to *Crotalus* venom.' *Toxicon*, 1: 5–18.

Russell, F. E., B. A. O'Brien and D. I. Inaba 1961 'Venoms and neuromuscular transmission.' *10th Pac. Sci. Congress*, 455.

Russell, F. E. and R. S. Scharffenberg 1964 'Bibliography of Snake Venoms and Venomous Snakes.' Bibliographies Associates, West Covina, Calif.

Tamiya, N., H. Arai and S. Sato 1967 'Studies on sea snake venoms: Crystallization of erabutoxins "a" and "b" from *Laticauda semifasciata* venom, and of Laticotoxin "a" from *Laticauda laticauda* venom.' *In*: Russell, F. E. and P. R. Saunders (eds.), *Animal Toxins*. p. 249, Pergamon Press, Oxford.

Vick, J. A., H. P. Ciuchta and E. H. Polley 1964 'Effect of snake venom and endotoxin on corticol electrical activity.' *Nature*, 203 : 1387.

Vick, J. A., H. P. Ciuchta and E. H. Polley 1965 'The effect of cobra venom on the respiratory mechanism of the dog.' *Arch. Int. Pharm.*, 153 : 424.

EFFECTS OF *VIPERA PALAESTINAE* HEMORRHAGIN ON BLOOD COAGULATION AND PLATELET FUNCTION

L. GROTTO, Z. JERUSHALMY and A. DE VRIES

Rogoff-Wellcome Medical Research Institute,
Tel-Aviv University Medical School, Beilinson Hospital,
Petah Tikva, Israel

SNAKE BITE HEMORRHAGE is primarily due to venom hemorrhagins, i.e. agents causing vessel wall damage, whereas coagulation disturbances may aggravate the bleeding. Hemorrhage is a prominent clinical sign of *Vipera palestinae* bite. Recently, a hemorrhagin was isolated from the venom of this snake in our laboratory (Grotto *et al.*, 1967). The purified hemorrhagin was found to possess a strong proteolytic activity, but its inhibition by diisopropyl fluorophosphate (DFP) or soybean trypsin inhibitor did not impair its ability to cause hemorrhage. It was therefore suggested that the vessel wall damaging principle is of a non-proteolytic nature (see also Ohsaka *et al.*, Volume I). The present study was undertaken to elucidate whether in addition to its vessel wall damaging activity, the hemorrhagin also affects blood coagulation or platelets.

Incubation of the hemorrhagin with human platelet-rich plasma at a concentration of 150 μg/ml caused prolongation of recalcification time and thrombin clotting time, accompanied by a reduction in the opacity and tensile strength of the clot. The hemorrhagin impaired also thromboplastin generation and yield, these effects being most evident when the hemorrhagin was preincubated with the plasma component; preincubation with platelets had almost no effect. On the other hand, preincubation with both plasma and platelets augmented the interference with thromboplastin generation.

In order to examine a possible action on fibrinogen, the hemorrhagin was incubated, in concentrations ranging from 100 to 240 $\mu g/ml$, with fibrinogen for varying periods of time. It was found that the hemorrhagin caused prolongation of thombin clotting time and decrease of clot opacity, these effects augmenting with incubation; after 16 hours incubation the fibrinogen became unclottable. DFP-treated hemorrhagin had no such effect.

The action of the hemorrhagin on fibrinogen caused a release of TCA-soluble peptides. However, this peptide release did not interfere with the ability of thrombin to further split off fibrinopeptides. It seems therefore that the bonds cleaved by the hemorrhagin in the fibrinogen are different from those susceptible to thrombin.

The fibrinogen degradation product obtained after incubation of fibrinogen with hemorrhagin had electrophoretic mobility and antigenic specificity similar to those of the intact molecule, as was established by acrylamide gel disc electrophoresis, gel diffusion and immunoelectrophoresis. This observation may be explained by limited proteolysis similar to that described by Alexander *et al.* (1966) for the initial stages of tryptic fibrinogen digestion, in which cleavage of one to two bonds already retarded the thrombin clotting kinetics; cleavage of 2 to 8 bonds finally rendered the fibrinogen unclottable by thrombin.

The interaction of thrombin with fibrinogen was impaired in the presence of hemorrhagin-treated fibrinogen. Clotting time was prolonged and the optical density of the clot was markedly diminished. This effect was shown to be due to the presence of the degraded fibrinogen and not to the presence of the TCA-soluble peptides.

Clots obtained from hemorrhagin-treated fibrinogen by thrombin-CaCl$_2$ mixture had diminished opacity and were soluble in urea. Hemorrhagin was furthermore found to inactivate the fibrin stabilizing factor (FSF). It is concluded therefore that the impairment of clot structure caused by the hemorrhagin is due to both its action on fibrinogen and FSF.

The hemorrhagin affected several platelet functions. Incubation of washed platelets with the hemorrhagin diminished their clot retracting activity; DFP-treated hemorrhagin had no such effect. ADP- and connective tissue-induced platelet aggregation were also affected by the hemorrhagin and so was connective tissue-induced release of platelet ADP. DFP-treated hemorrhagin interfered only partially with these platelet functions. Platelet factor 3 availability and platelet factor 4 release were not affected by the hemorrhagin.

The *in vivo* effect of the hemorrhagin was studied in guinea pigs. Intra-cardial injection of 1 LD_{50} of the hemorrhagin (150 μg/250 gm body weight) resulted in widespread hemorrhages and marked hypofibrinogenemia; the drop in fibrinogen level ranged from 40 to 70 per cent. Clotting time, clot retraction and platelet count were almost unaffected. DFP-treated hemorr-hagin produced hemorrhages as well but did not cause a significant hypo-fibrinogenemia. It is pointed out that the concentration of hemorrhagin needed to obtain demonstrable effects on clotting and fibrinogen in vitro exceeded by far that estimated to occur in the circulating blood following administration of one LD_{50}. These observations support the assumption that the hemorrhagic effect of *Vipera palaestinae* hemorrhagin is primarily due to its action on the vessel wall. An aggravating role of the proteolytic activity of the hemorrhagin can, however, not be excluded.

In conclusion: *Vipera palaestinae* hemorrhagin was shown to have diverse effects on the blood coagulation process in vitro—impairing thrombin form-ation, fibrinogen clottability, FSF activity and various platelet functions. These effects were more evident after incubation of the hemorrhagin with the various substrates. 'Instantaneous' action of the hemorrhagin was manifested only in diminished opacity of the clot and impairment of platelet aggregation. Treatment of the hemorrhagin with DFP abolished almost all these activities except for a partial effect on platelet aggregation and connective tissue-induced platelet ADP release. It is therefore assumed that the disturbances of the coagulation process and platelet function induced by the hemorrhagin are mainly due to its proteolytic activity. Administration of hemorrhagin to guinea pigs caused widespread hemorrhages associated with moderate hypo-fibrinogenemia. DFP-treated hemorrhagin caused hemorrhage without significant hypofibrinogenemia.

References

Alexander, B., A. Rimon and E. Katchalsky 1966 'Action of water insoluble trypsin derivatives on fibrinogen clottability.' *Thromb. Diath. Haemorrh.* (Stuttg.), 16: 507.

Grotto, L., Ch. Moroz, A. de Vries and N. Goldblum 1967 'Isolation of *Vipera palaestinae* hemorrhagin and distinction between its hemorrhagic and proteolytic activities.' *Biochim. Biophys. Acta*, 133: 356.

DISSOCIATION BETWEEN HEMORRHAGIC, ENZYMATIC AND LETHAL ACTIVITY OF SOME SNAKE VENOMS AND OF BEE VENOM AS STUDIED IN A NEW MODEL

I. L. BONTA, N. BHARGAVA and B. B. VARGAFTIG

*Department of Pharmacology, Medical Faculty Rotterdam,
The Netherlands; Organon Research Laboratories,
Eragny-Sur-Epte, France and Oss, The Netherlands*

INTRODUCTION

MANY STUDIES have been devoted to the hemorrhagic activity of snake venoms, and these have been included in a recent review (Jiminez-Porras, 1968). At the outset it is debatable which components of the snake venoms have hemorrhagic activity, what is the mechanism of this activity and which drugs can counteract the hemorrhages produced by the venoms. The uncertainty is evident when one considers that separated fractions of the venoms were seldomly tested for hemorrhagic activity, and the biological methods for testing were neither sensitive enough nor sufficiently reproducible.

In the model which we developed to study the hemorrhagic properties of snake venoms we chose the lung as our test object, because this organ has a rich vascularization. We have used the dog lung in open-thorax preparations and have shown that the surface of the lung is particularly suitable for the assessment of topical hemorrhagic effects of vasculotoxic venoms or their fractions (Bonta *et al.*, 1965, 1969a, 1970). The method, however, was unsuitable to investigate a dissociation between the hemorrhagic and lethal effects. We therefore introduced another technique, which consists of injecting the venoms intrathoracally in mice. This method enabled us to simultaneously determine the pulmonary hemorrhagic effect, behaviour change and lethality caused by venoms and their fractions.

MATERIALS AND METHODS

Materials

Naja naja, Agkistrodon piscivorus and *Apis mellifica* (honey bee) venoms were obtained from commercial sources. The various fractions of the venoms were prepared by gel filtration on Sephadex columns and the optical density was measured as described in a previous paper (Bhargava *et al.*, 1970). The heparin used was a commercial batch (Thromboliquine[R]). For injection all materials were dissolved in Sörensen phosphate buffer (pH 7.38). All solutions were freshly prepared before use.

Enzymatic and hemolytic activity

BAEE-ase activity was studied under the conditions described by Kraut and Bhargava (1963). Phospholipase A activity was determined by the method of Doizaki (1964). Estimation of hemolysis was carried out according to a procedure published in a previous paper by Bhargava *et al.* (1970).

Dog lung-surface hemorrhage test

Open-thorax preparations were made of anaesthetized dogs. Filter paper discs of 5 mm diameter were soaked in solutions of the venoms or their fractions and applied to the lung surface for 3 minutes. Circumscribed bleedings were thus evoked. The large surface of the dog lung permitted the production of 15–20 hemorrhagic spots and it was possible to establish the qualitative character, the onset and the intensity of the micro-circulatory lesions. Details of the method were published previously by Bonta *et al.* (1970).

Mouse pulmonary hemorrhage test

Male albino mice (19–21 gm) purchased from the TNO Animal Centre were used in groups of 5–10. The venoms or their fractions were administered intrathoracally using tuberculine-syringes fitted with a specially constructed needle having a tip of 1.5 mm length. The injected materials thus reached the intrapleural space or the pulmonary surface rather than deeper parts in the lungs. The site of injection was the lower right quarter of the chest, and the volume administered was 0.1 ml/10 gm body weight, though occasionally 0.5 ml/10 gm was administered. The animals were observed for behaviour alterations and the survival time was recorded to the nearest second. Animals surviving two hours were sacrificed by ether. From all mice the lungs were removed for inspection of hemorrhages. Additionally the lungs were weighed and a lung index (= $\frac{\text{lung weight}}{\text{body weight}} \times 100$) calculated. It was considered that an increase in the lung index is an indication of the increased lung weight as a consequence of local blood extravasation. In most experiments the venoms or the fractions were administered in a dose of 7.5 mg/kg (= 150 μg/mouse). Pilot experiments showed that this dose of *N. naja* venom produced pronounced hemorrhage and a markedly increased lung index. Subsequently we observed that 7.5 mg/kg produced a supramaximal increase of the lung index. Accordingly, in some experiments a lower dose chosen from a logarithmic scale was administered. In a further series of experiments the mice were pretreated by intrathoracally administered heparin. Control mice received an intrathoracal injection of 0.1 ml/10 gm phosphate buffer (pH 7.38).

RESULTS AND DISCUSSION

N. naja venom and bee venom when applied to the dog lung surface produced identical diffuse types of bleedings. The hemorrhages caused by *A. piscivorus* venom, however, had dotted (petechial) appearance. With high doses of *A. piscivorus* venom the petechiae fused, and dark spots (microthrombi?) appeared in the centre of the hemorrhagic spot. The bleedings thus produced by the venoms were strictly dose dependent with respect to onset and intensity (Bonta *et al.*, 1970). It was also shown that *A. piscivorus* venom displayed two to three times the hemorrhagic potency of *N. naja* venom. It appears that bee venom is approximately half as potent as *N. naja* venom. More exact figures for the hemorrhagic potency of bee venom, however, are still to be obtained from dose-response experiments.

The dropwise addition of heparin (50 mg/ml) to solutions of *N. naja*, *A. piscivorus* and bee venom produced a visible precipitate. After centrifugation the supernatant of the heparinized *N. naja* venom was practically devoid of

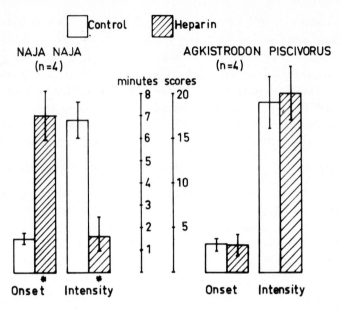

FIGURE 1.   Effect of heparin on the hemorrhagic activity of two snake venoms as tested on the dog lung surface.

Mean values ± SE. Number of observations in brackets. Significant results are marked with asterisk, P < 0.025

hemorrhagic activity on the canine lung surface, as shown by the fact that the onset of the bleedings was very much prolonged and the intensity was drastically reduced. The hemorrhagic effect of heparinized *A. piscivorus* venom remained undiminished or was occasionally slightly enhanced (Figure 1). Heparinization of the bee venom resulted in a similar abolition of hemorrhagic activity as was the case with *N. naja* venom. Heating of *N. naja* venom at pH 5.5 for 15 minutes at 100° C did not appreciably reduce the hemorrhagic effect, but the same producedure at pH 8 entirely abolished this activity.

The above results were presented in greater detail in previous papers (Bonta *et al.*, 1969a, 1970; Bhargava *et al.*, 1970), and they indicate that the main vasculotoxic component of *N. naja* venom and of bee venom is possibly a material having similar chemical properties as the Direct Lytic Factor.

The venom fractions obtained by gel filtration were investigated in the dog lung-surface method and in the mouse pulmonary-hemorrhage test. The results obtained with the canine lung were published previously (Bhargava *et*

TABLE 1   Dissociation of enzymatic, hemorrhagic and toxic effects of venoms and their fractions

Material tested	Molecular weight	In vitro activity			Hemorrhage on lung of dogs and mice	Systemic effect in mice*	
		BAEE-ase % (100% by 10 µg trypsin)	Phospholipase turbidimetric units	Hemolysis % by 10 µg material		Behaviour	Lethality
Naja naja crude venom		0	2.89	4.5	+++	Respir. failure	+++[3]
G 50 III	< 10.000	0	1.68	4.5	+++	Respir. failure	+++[3]
A. piscivorus crude venom		50	10.80	3.3	+++	Sedation	++[4]
G 50 I	> 10.000	86	0	0	+[1]	No effect	non lethal[5]
G 50 II	~ 10.000	58	0	0	0	Sedation	non lethal[5]
G 50 III	< 10.000	0	8.72	0	+++	Sedation	non lethal[5]
Apis mellifica crude venom		0	9.95	97	+++	Delayed respir. failure	++[4]
G 50 II	~ 10.000	0	18.88	0	++[2]	Sedation	non lethal[5]
G 50 III A	5.000	0	0	98	+++	Rigid gait	++[4]
G 50 III B	? 5.000	0	0	77.5	+++	Sedation	++[4]
G 25 II	< 5.000	0	0	?	+++	Sedation	non lethal[5]
Melittin	2.600	?	?	?	+++	Sedation	non lethal[5]
Apamin	< 2.000	?	?	?	0	Convulsion	non lethal[5]

*) 7.5 mg/kg intrathoracally
? in vitro activity not tested by us
1) inactive in mice
2) inactive in dogs
3) survival < 10 minutes
4) survival 10 < 60 minutes
5) survival 2 hours or more

al., 1970). There was clear evidence that the hemorrhagic effect of *N. naja, A. piscivorus* and *Apis mellifica* venom was confined to fractions having a molecular weight of less than 10,000. This observation was confirmed in the recent studies on mice. The properties of the various fractions are shown in Table 1. In this table the hemorrhagic activities were observed either on dog lungs or in mice and are presented in a single column. The same venom fractions which showed pronounced vasculotoxic effects on canine lungs, displayed hemorrhagic effects also in mice. The G 50 II fraction of bee venom produced a delay in the onset of hemorrhage (1—2 hours after application) in mice and was not hemorrhagic in dogs. With the canine lung method however the observation was terminated 15 minutes after the topical application.

It can be seen from Table 1 that the hemorrhagic activity is not necessarily associated with phospholipase, BAEE-ase or hemolytic activity of the venoms. The hemorrhagic G 50 III fraction of *N. naja* venom showed low phospholipase and low hemolytic activity. The low degree of hemolysis found by us with *N. naja* venom is in agreement with observations by others (Slotta *et al.*, 1967). The main hemorrhagic fraction of bee venom (G 50 IIIB, from which the subfraction G 25 II was separated) was devoid of phospholipase activity, but displayed high hemolytic activity. The G 50 IIIB fraction possibly contained a high proportion of melittin, which was also found to produce lung hemorrhage in mice. The hemorrhagic component of *A. piscivorus* venom (G 50 III) showed high phospholipase but no hemolytic activity. None of the hemorrhagic fractions showed BAEE-ase activity. All this evidence is in agreement with earlier findings showing that the potent BAEE-splitting enzymes trypsin or pancreatic kallikrein and purified phospholipase A are unable to produce hemorrhages in pulmonary vessels (Bonta *et al.*, 1969a). It was also proven that Trasylol, a natural inhibitor of proteases and esterases, was without effect on the hemorrhagic activity of either of the venoms studied (Bonta *et al.*, 1969b). On the other hand Tu *et al.* (1967) found a correlation between hemorrhagic activity and TAME-hydrolysing capacity of venoms. Further studies are needed to explain the possible connection between the findings of Tu and the observation that some enzyme inhibitors (benzamidine, DFP, EDTA) reduced venom hemorrhagic activity (Bonta *et al.*, 1969b).

The study of a relatively narrow dose range of intrathoracally administered *N. naja* venom in mice has shown that increase in lung weight and survival time had a reciprocal relationship. The increase in lung weight came close to maximal with the lowest dose tested (Figure 2). The dose of 7.5 mg/kg,

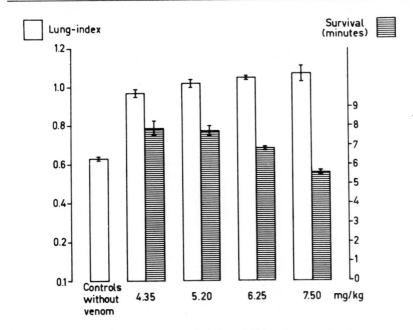

FIGURE 2.   Effect of intrathoracally administered *Naja naja* venom in mice.
Mean values ± SE of groups of 6 mice each. For explanation of lung index see Materials and Methods

which caused death in 5—6 minutes, produced appreciable hemorrhage and lung weight increase as early as 1 minute after the administration (Figure 3). The lung weight increased steadily after injection and in mice succumbing to the venom the lungs showed nearly double the weight as compared to mice without venom treatment. At the time of writing this paper the histological examination of the lungs was not completed, hence no information is available showing to what extent blood extravasation or pulmonary congestion was the contributive factor to lung weight increase.

When heparinized *N. naja* venom was administered to mice, the lungs were neither hemorrhagic, nor was there an appreciable gain in the lung-index. The survival time of the mice treated with heparinized venom was approximately twice as long as that of mice receiving venom to which no heparin had been added. Also it can be seen from Table 2 that there was little difference as to whether the venom was administered immediately after the addition of heparin, or the heparin-venom mixture was incubated and centrifuged prior

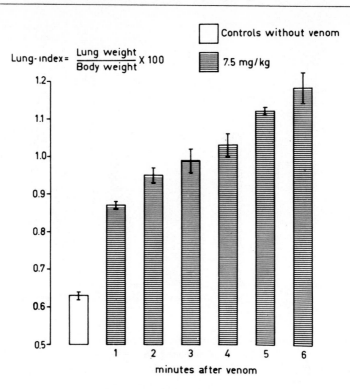

FIGURE 3.   Time course of lung-index change in mice by intrathoracally administered *Naja naja* venom.

Mean values ± SE of separate groups, which were sacrificed at various time points following the administration of venom. Groups of 6 mice

to injection. This indicates the speed of the process by which heparin forms an inactive complex with the strongly basic vasculotoxic component of *N. naja* venom.

Subsequent experiments have shown that protection towards pulmonary hemorrhage was achieved when the mice were treated intrathoracally with heparin (Figure 4). As the heparin was administered at the same site where the venom was to be injected, inactive-complex formation may have occurred at the injection site. Heparin, however, provided protection to the mice when administered as long as 3–6 hours before the venom was injected; hence, it is not inconceivable that heparin, after being absorbed, may have protected the capillaries by some as yet unknown mechanism. It was proposed that snake venom-induced hemorrhages occur by an action on the perivascular inter-

TABLE 2   Alteration of the effects of *Naja naja* venom by addition of heparin Groups of 10 mice. Intrathoracal injection.

Addition to venom solution	Manipulation before injection	Material tested	Surviving time, minutes	Lung index	Hemorrhage on lung
—	—	phosphate buffer	sacrificed	0.64 ± 0.01	—
—	—	*N. naja* venom (7.5 mg/kg)	6'14" ± 0'05"	1.09 ± 0.02	pronounced
Heparin 1.3 mg[1] to each 1 mg venom	—	*N. naja* venom (7.5 mg/kg) Heparin (10 mg/kg) }[3]	11'08" ± 0'57"	0.76 ± 0.02	—
Heparin 1.3 mg to each 1 mg venom[1]	Incubation and centrifugation 1000 g	Supernatant[2]	9'45" ± 0'17"	0.87 ± 0.02	—
Heparin (50 mg/ml) dropwise, until visible precipitation	Centrifugation 10,000 g	Supernatant[2]	13'45" ± 0'18"	0.77 ± 0.02	—

1) clear solution.
2) volume adjusted to inject an equivalent of 7.5 mg/kg venom dose.
3) group of 6 mice.

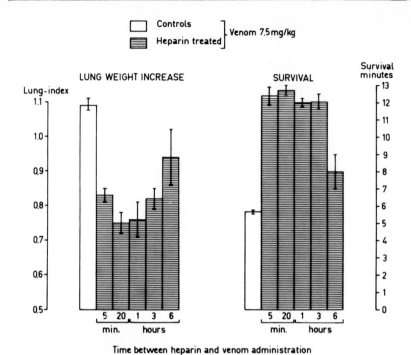

FIGURE 4.   *Naja naja* venom effect in heparin treated mice.
Heparin was administered intrathoracally in a dose of 10 mg/kg. The venom dose, also intrathoracally administered, was 7.5 mg/kg. Mean values ± SE of groups of 6 mice

cellular ground substance (de Vries *et al.*, 1962), largely composed of acid mucopolysaccharides. Heparin protection of perivascular tissue from noxious influences has not yet been studied.

In vitro precipitation of the *N. naja* venom-vasculotoxin by heparin resulted in a doubled survival time in mice, but did not prevent death. No mortality occurred however when the animals were treated by venom which was heated at pH 8 prior to injection (Table 3). These experiments indicate that the heparin-precipitable, strongly basic vasculotoxin of *N. naja* venom contributes little to the lethal effect of the venom. Heating at pH 8 however destroys not only the hemorrhagic factor, but the lethal component of the venom as well. It appears from a recent study that the main toxin in *N. naja* venom is a glycoprotein (Braganca and Patel, 1965).

TABLE 3   The dissociation of *Naja naja* venom into two lethal components. The equivalent of 7.5 mg/kg venom was administered intrathoracally to each group of 5–10 mice.

Manipulation before injection	Surviving time, minutes	Lung index	Hemorrhage on lung
—	6'03" ± 0'09"	1.10 ± 0.03	pronounced
pH 5.6, heating at 100° C, 15 min	8'18" ± 0'11"	1.04 ± 0.04	pronounced
pH 8.0, heating at 100° C, 15 min	> 2 hours*)	0.68 ± 0.02	—
Heparin precipitation, centrifugation 10,000 g	13'45" ± 0'18"	0.77 ± 0.02	—

*) After 2 hours sacrificed to inspect and weigh the lungs

SUMMARY

The hemorrhagic actions of venoms and their fractions obtained by gel-filtration were studied by topical application on the lung surface of dogs and intrathoracal administration in mice. Similar type of hemorrhages were caused by the venoms of *Naja naja* and *Apis mellifica*, whereas the bleedings by *Agkistrodon piscivorus* showed a different appearance. The hemorrhagic action of all three venoms was confined to components having a molecular weight of less than 10,000. No correlation was found between the hemorrhagic effect and phospholipase, BAEE-ase or hemolytic activity of the venoms.

Heparin forms an inactive complex with the vasculotoxic components of *N. naja* and *A. mellifica* venom. The hemorrhagic activity of *A. piscivorus* venom remained unaffected by the addition of heparin.

Intrathoracally administered heparin in mice provided complete protection towards the topical hemorrhagic action of *N. naja* venom. The survival of the heparin-treated mice was prolonged, but they were not protected from the lethal effect of the venom. Heating at pH 8 destroys the vasculotoxic and the lethal component of *N. naja* venom. The main lethal factor in *N. naja* venom is unlikely to be identical with the heparin-precipitable vasculotoxic component.

ACKNOWLEDGMENTS

Thanks are given to Mrs. K. de Vries for devoted assistance during this work. Melittin was obtained by courtesy of Prof. E. Habermann (Giessen) and Apamin was supplied by Prof. J. F. Arens (Utrecht). We are indebted to Mr. D. W. R. Hall for linguistic correction of the text.

References

Bhargava, N., P. Zirinis, I. L. Bonta and B. B. Vargaftig 1970 'Comparison of hemorrhagic factors of the venoms of *Naja naja*, *Agkistrodon piscivorus* and *Apis mellifera.' Biochem. Pharmacol.* **19**: 2405.

Bonta, I. L., N. Bhargava and B. B. Vargaftig 1969b 'Hemorrhagic snake venoms and kallikrein inhibitors as tools to study factors determining the integrity of the vessel wall.' *In*: Sicuteri, F. and M. Rocha E. Silva (eds.), *Proceedings of International Symposium on cardiovascular and neuro-actions of Bradykinin and related kinins, Fiesole*, p. 19. Plenum Press.

Bonta, I. L., C. J. de Vos and A. Delver 1965 'Inhibitory effects of estriol-16, 17-disodium succinate on local haemorrhages induced by snake venom in canine heart-lung preparations.' *Acta Endocrinol.*, **48** : 137.

Bonta, I. L., B. B. Vargaftig, N. Bhargava and C. J. de Vos 1970 'Method for study of snake venom induced haemorrhages.' *Toxicon*, **8** : 3.

Bonta, I. L., B. B. Vargaftig, C. J. de Vos and H. Grijsen 1969a 'Haemorrhagic mechanisms of some snake venoms in relation to protection by estriol succinate of blood vessel damage.' *Life Sci.*, **8**: 881.

Braganca, B. M. and N. T. Patel 1965 'Glycoproteins as components of the lethal factors in cobra venom (*Naja naja*).' *Can. J. Biochem.*, **43**: 915.

De Vries, A., E. Condrea, C. Klibansky, J. Rechnic, C. Moroz and C. Kirschmann 1962 'Hematological effects of the venoms of two Near Eastern snakes: *Vipera palestinae* and *Echis colorata.' New Istanbul Contrib. Clin. Sci.*, **5**: 151. Cited by Jimenez-Porras, J. M. 1968 *In*: Ann. Rev. Pharmacol., 8, 299.

Doizaki, W. M. 1964 'Turbidimetric assay for phospholipase A.' *J. Lab. Clin. Med.*, **3**: 524.

Jimenez-Porras, J. M. 1968 'Pharmacology of peptides and proteins in snake venoms.' *Ann. Rev. Pharmacol.*, **8**: 299.

Kraut, H. and N. Bhargava 1963 'Verhalten des Kallikreins Inaktivators gegenüber Fermenten–II.' *Hoppe-Seyler's Z. Physiol. Chem.*, **334** : 236.

Slotta, K. H., J. D. Gonzalez and S. C. Roth 1967 'The direct and indirect hemolytic factors from animal venoms.' **In**: Russell, F.E. and P.R. Saunders (eds.), *Animal Toxins*, p. 369. Pergamon Press, Oxford.

Tu, A. T., P. M. Toom and S. Ganthavorn 1967 'Hemorrhagic and proteolytic activities of Thailand snake venoms.' *Biochem. Pharmacol.*, **16** : 2125.

ROLE OF BRADYKININ IN THE FATAL SHOCK INDUCED BY *BOTHROPS JARARACA* VENOM IN THE RAT

A. M. ROTHSCHILD and J. A. ALMEIDA*

Department of Pharmacology, Faculty of Medicine of Ribeirao Preto,
Brazil

BRADYKININ and related kinin are a group of peptides, originating from plasma α_2-globulins, which in view of their powerful vaso-dilating and vascular permeability-increasing actions are able to cause strong hypotension in animals and man. The ability to release bradykinin is being found in an increasing number of animal venoms including those of *Bothrops jararaca* (Rocha e Silva *et al.*, 1949), several crotalic and bothropic species (Deutsch and Diniz, 1955), *Agkistrodon halys blomhoffii* (Sato *et al.*, 1965), *Heloderma suspectum* (Mebs, 1969), *Echis colorata* (Cohen *et al.*, 1970) and *Vipera xanthina palestinae* (Rothschild and Rothschild, unpublished).

Many of the bradykinin-releasing venoms are also powerful blood-coagulating agents; intravascular clotting has been considered as the cause of death following the innoculation of sufficiently high doses of these, so-called 'coagulating venoms' (Grasset and Schwartz, 1954; Boquet, 1960).

In the present work kinin release and lethality caused by *Bothrops jararaca* venom were studied in rats in which the blood coagulating effect of the venom had been suppressed by suitable preliminary treatments.

MATERIALS AND METHODS

Male, Wistar rats, weighing 250–300 g were employed.

---

* Research Fellow, State Research Foundation (FAPESP) Sao Paulo, Brazil.

Drugs

Heparin (Roche); Cellulose sulfate, prepared according to Astrup *et al.*, (1944). *Bothrops jararaca* venom from Instituto Butantan, Brazil. Polybrene from Abbot Labs., Chicago. Bradykinin triacetate from Sandoz (Basle). All materials were injected intravenously through the venous sinus of the penis of ether-anesthetized animals.

Blood pressure was measured in the carotid artery using a mercury manometer.

Samples of blood were obtained by cardiac puncture. Bradykinin levels in oxalated plasma were determined according to Diniz and Carvalho (1963). Clotting times were measured by the Lee-White technique. Fibrinogen in plasma was determined according to Reiner and Cheung (1959); in some samples, prior to the addition of thrombin, Polybrene (200 μg/ml) was added to neutralize heparin or cellulose sulfate. This procedure did not alter the amount of fibrinogen found and was subsequently omitted.

RESULTS

The first part of Table 1 shows the effects on survival time, plasma bradykini-nogen and *in-vitro* clotting time of the blood of rats receiving increasing doses of *Bothrops jararaca* venom intravenously. At the rapidly fatal dose of 2 mg/kg, the venom induced the disappearance of 2/3 of the animals' circulat-ing bradykininogen as well as a considerable shortening of its blood clotting time. This event, which became nearly instantaneous in drawn blood, was followed by rapid clot lysis. This picture was not substantially changed in animals which had received, 1 mg (100 units)/kg of heparin, 15 min prior to the injection of venom, a dose which inhibits the coagulation of normal rat blood. When the dose of heparin was doubled, marked changes in the effects of subsequently administered *Bothrops* venom were observed. Not only was complete protection from death obtained, but also no clotting of drawn blood was observed. Bradykininogen disappearance on the other hand was as extensive as in the control animals.

A lethal dose of Bothrops venom evoked rapid circulatory collapse in the rat (Figure 1(a)). In the heparin-protected animal, the venom still evoked a rapidly progressing, intense hypotension which was however overcome by the animal after 10–15 min. (Figure 1(b)).

TABLE 1   Effect of heparin (Hep) and of cellulose sulfate (CS) on mortality, plasma bradykininogen (BKG) and the clotting time of the blood of rats injected with *B. jararaca* venom (Vb)

Treatment mg/kg, i.v.	Survival time	BKG* %	Clotting time (Lee-White)
Saline		100	60 sec
Vb, 0.5	> 7 days	65	15 sec[ly]
Vb, 1.0	14 min	40	10 sec[ly]
Vb, 2.0	3 min	33	10 sec[ly]
Hep, 1.0		100	> 2 h
Hep, 2.0		100	> 2 h
Hep, 1.0 ;after 15'Vb, 2.0	8 min	35	10 sec
Hep, 2.0; after 15'Vb, 2.0	> 7 days	33	> 2 h
CS, 1.0	> 7 days	53	62 sec
CS, 1.0;after 15'Vb, 2.0	> 7 days	21	> 2 h

* Det. 3−5 min after treatment ;controls had 4.8 ± 0.2 units BKG/ml.
ly indicates clotting followed by rapid lysis.
Each result is the average of 3−6 experiments.

Cellulose sulfate is an anionic polysaccharide capable of causing the release of kinin and the partial disappearance of bradykininogen from rat plasma *in-vivo* and *in vitro* (Rothschild, 1968, Rothschild and Gascon, 1966). The last part of Table 1 shows that cellulose sulfate caused a fall of 50% of the animals' plasma bradykininogen without affecting blood clotting time. Treated animals were resistant to the lethal effect of subsequently administered *Bothrops* venom; upon envenomation, they showed a further loss of plasma bradykininogen but also an abolition of the hypercoagulative effect of the venom. Figure 2 shows that cellulose sulfate caused a marked, yet transitory fall of blood pressure; as previously shown (Rothschild, 1968), this is due to the release of bradykinin. Subsequently injected *Bothrops* venom caused a renewed fall of blood pressure; this effect was overcome by the animal which became desensitized to the hypotensive effects of both *Bothrops* venom and cellulose sulfate.

The effect of heparin on the clotting ability of *Bothrops jararaca* venom was also investigated *in vitro* using rat blood containing these agents at the approximate concentration in which they initially existed in the treated animals; a value of 80 ml of blood/kg body weight was assumed. Table 2

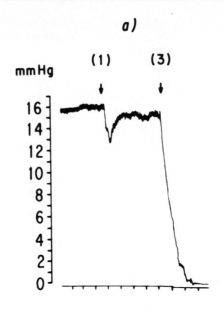

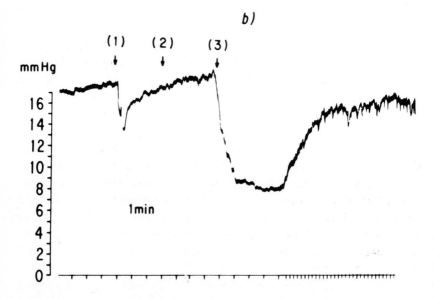

FIGURE 1.   Effect of *Bothrops jararaca* venom on the blood pressure of (a) normal and (b) heparin-treated rats. At (1), Bradykinin, 1 μg; (2), Heparin, 2 mg/kg; (3), *Bothrops* venom, 2 mg/kg

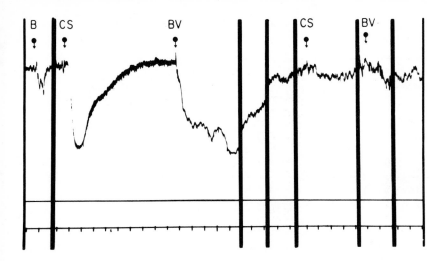

FIGURE 2.   Effect of *Bothrops jararaca* venom on the blood pressure of cellulose sulfate-treated rat. At B, bradykinin, 1 μg; CS, cellulose sulfate, 1 mg/kg; BV, *Bothrops* venom, 2 mg/kg. Dark bands: 5 min stopping period of kymograph drum

TABLE 2   Effect of the *in vitro* addition of *Bothrops jararaca* venom (BV) and of heparin (Hep) on the clotting time of rat blood

Addition (μg/ml)	Clotting Time (sec)	
	Normal Blood	Oxalated blood
—	59	inc.
BV, 25	14	42
Hep, 25	inc.	—
Hep + BV	209	564

inc: blood incoagulable for more than 2 h. Each result is the average of 3 determinations.

shows that *Bothrops* venom markedly shortened the clotting time of both normal and oxalated blood. Heparin retarded this effect to a marked extent in both cases.

In contrast to heparin-treated rats, cellulose sulfate-treated animals had normal blood clotting times before being given the venom. Other reasons for the protective effect of the sulfopolysaccharide were therefore sought for.

TABLE 3   Effect of cellulose sulfate (CS) and of heparin on the fibrinogen content of the plasma of the rat

Treatment mg/kg (i.v.)	Fibrinogen mg% ± S.E.M.		P
	Controls	Treated	
Saline	246 ± 14	238 ± 12	n.s.
CS, 1.0	205 ± 10	57 ± 15	< 0.05
Hep, 2.0	194 ± 10	184 ± 9	n.s.

Blood samples were collected 5 min following treatment.
Each result is the average of 5 experiments.

Table 3 shows that cellulose sulfate effectively lowered the plasma fibrinogen levels of the rat.

DISCUSSION

The results presented in this paper indicate that among the three major hematological alterations produced by *B. jararaca* venom in the rat i.e., hypercoagulability, enhanced fibrinolytic activity and plasma bradykininogen loss, the first one is the most probable cause of acute death. This is shown by the full protection offered by heparin at a dose which failed to prevent the bradykininogen destroying action of the venom while neutralizing its hyper-coagulant effect.

If it is assumed that all the bradykininogen destroyed by the venom is converted into bradykinin, a discharge of 1.5–2 μg of this polypeptide per ml of plasma must have occurred in the envenomed animals. Although causing marked hypotension, this release was tolerated by the heparin-treated animal. This tolerance is probably due to the rapid binding and destruction of brady-kinin by the animal's own tissues (Ferreira and Vane, 1967), as well as by its destruction by peptidases from *Bothrops* venom itself (Rocha e Silva *et al.*, 1949).

As shown by the *in vitro* results, *Bothrops* venom enhanced the speed of clotting of both normal and of oxalated rat blood though to a different extent in each case. This indicates that besides its 'thrombinic' action, the venom also potentiates earlier phases of the clotting process. In view of its protective efficiency, heparin must be able to counteract the 'thrombinic' action of the venom. Whether it also affects its other clotting effects remains to be investigated.

Like heparin, cellulose sulfate afforded protection to the rat without preventing the hypotensive and bradykininogen-destroying action of subsequently administered *Bothrops* venom. Unlike heparin however, cellulose sulfate at the dose employed, had little effect on blood clotting time. Its protective action is most probably due to its strong fibrinogenopenic effect. This effect, which is much more pronounced *in vivo* than *in vitro* (unpublished results), is probably largely due to the enzymatic removal of fibrinogen from the circulation by cellulose sulfate-activated fibrinolysin (Rosa, 1969).

Cellulose sulfate-induced fibrinogenopenia leading to the disappearance of 3/4 of the animal's circulatory fibrinogen, could make venom-induced intravascular clotting a tolerable phenomenon. Clots, if formed, would be tenuous and probably quickly dissolved by the fibrinolytic activity induced by cellulose sulfate as well as by the venom itself.

Cellulose sulfate has been shown to be a useful tool for the study of the role of bradykinin in cutaneous anaphylaxis (Rothschild, 1968a) and endotoxin shock (Rothschild and Castania, 1968). By preventing the death of experimental animals this, as well as other sulfopolysaccharides, could become useful tools for the study of pharmacological effects of large, otherwise lethal doses of venoms or their components.

SUMMARY

Heparin or cellulose sulfate protects rats from death caused by intravenous injection of *Bothrops jararaca* venom. Heparin did not prevent the breakdown of plasma bradykinin precursor (bradykininogen) by the venom, but effectively counteracted its hypercoagulative action.

Cellulose sulfate caused extensive plasma bradykininogen consumption, did not alter blood coagulation time but led to marked fibrinogenopenia. This effect is probably the cause of the protection afforded by this sulfopolysaccharide.

It is concluded that even a massive release of bradykinin by *Bothrops jararaca* venom can be well tolerated by rats provided that intravascular coagulation is prevented by a suitable treatment.

References

Astrup, T., B. Galsmar and M. Volkert 1944 'Polysaccharide sulfuric acids as anti-coagulants.' *Acta Physiol. Scand.*, 8: 215–221.

Boquet, P. 1968 'Pharmacology and Toxicology of Snake Venoms of Europe and the Mediterranean Regions.' *In*: Bucherl W., E. Buckley and V. Deulofeu, (eds.), *Venomous Animals and their Venoms*. Vol. I Academic Press, New York.

Cohen, I., M. Zur, E. Kaminski and A. de Vries 1970 'Isolation and characterization of kinin-releasing enzymes of *Echis coloratus* venom' (In press).

Deutsch, H. F. and C. R. Diniz 1955 'Some proteolytic activity of snake venoms.' *J. Biol. Chem.*, 216: 17.

Diniz, C. R. and I. F. Carvalho 1963 'A micro-method for determination of bradykinin-ogen under several conditions.' *Ann. N.Y. Acad. Sci.*, 104: 77–89.

Ferreira, S. H. and J. R. Vane 1967 'The disappearance of bradykinin and eledoisin in the circulation and vascular beds of the cat.' *Brit. J. Pharmacol.*, 30: 417.

Grasset, E. and D. E. Schwartz 1954 'Inhibition des principes coagulants de venins de serpents par le sulfate de dextrane.' *Path. u. Bakteriol.*, 17: 38.

Mebs, D. 1969 'Isolierung und Eigenschaften eines Kallikreins aus dem Gift der Kruste-nechse *Heloderma suspectum.*' *Hoppe-Seyler's Z. Physiol. Chem.*, 350: 821.

Reiner, M. and H. L. Cheung 1959 'A practical method for the determination of fibrin-ogen.' *Clin. Chem.*, 5: 414.

Rocha e Silva, M., W. T. Beraldo and G. Rosenfeld 1949 'Bradykinin, a hypotensive and smooth muscle stimulating factor released from plasma globulin by snake venoms and trypsin.' *Am. J. Physiol.*, 156: 261.

Rosa, A. T. 1969 'On the Fibrinolytic Activity Evoked by Cellulose Sulfate in Rat Plasma.' Ph.D. Dissertation. School of Pharmacy of Ribeirao Preto, Brazil.

Rothschild, A. M. 1968 'Pharmacodynamic properties of cellulose sulphate, a bradykininogen-depleting agent in the rat.' *Brit. J. Pharmacol.*, 35: 501.

Rothschild, A. M. 1968a 'Role of anaphylatoxin and of bradykinin in passive cutaneous anaphylaxis against heterologous precipitating antibody in the rat.' *In: Symposium on Immunopharmacology*, London, 11 83. Pergamon Press, Oxford.

Rothschild, A. M. and L. A. Gascon 1966 'Sulphuric esters of polysaccharides as activators of a bradykinin-forming system in plasma.' *Nature*, 212: 1364.

Rothschild, A. M. and A. Castania 1968 'Endotoxin shock in dogs pretreated with cellulose sulphate, an agent causing partial plasma kininogen depletion.' *J. Pharm. Pharmacol.*, 20: 77.

Sato, T., S. Iwanaga, Y. Mizushima and T. Suzuki 1965 'Studies on snake venoms. XV. Separation of arginine ester hydrolase of *Agkistrodon halys blomhoffii* into three enzymatic entities: "Bradykinin releasing", "clotting" and "permeability increasing". *J. Biochem.*, 47: 380.

THE EFFECT OF SCORPION VENOM ON BLOWFLY LARVAE

E. ZLOTKIN[1], G. FRAENKEL[2], F. MIRANDA[3], S. LISSITZKY[3] and A. SHULOV[1]

[1]*Department of Entomology and Venomous Animals, Hebrew University, Jerusalem, Israel,* [2] *Department of Entomology, University of Illinois, Urbana, Ill., U. S. A. and* [3]*Laboratoire de Biochimie Médicale, Faculté de Médecine, Marseille, France*

BECAUSE OF THE MEDICAL IMPORTANCE of scorpion venoms, mammals have hitherto served as the major test animals for pharmacological investigations. The lethality test on mice was used as the usual criterion for estimating venom potency and for purifying the venom's neurotoxic components (Lissitzky *et al.*, 1956; Miranda, 1964; Miranda *et al.*, 1964a, 1964b, 1966; Rochat, 1964; Watt, 1964; Gomez and Diniz, 1966; Rochat *et al.*, 1967).

On the other hand it should be stressed that in nature venom of scorpions serves to paralyze arthropods (mainly insects), their natural prey and food (Bearg, 1961). Thus we thought it interesting to compare the relative potency of scorpion venom in a mammal and an insect, and to investigate the chemical basis of these activities. From this point of view a study of the response of *Sarcophaga argyrostoma* fleshfly larvae to scorpion venom was undertaken.

Injection of a solution of scorpion venom into a fly larva causes a quick and immediate contraction of the body accompanied by a complete paralysis (Figure 1). The duration and rate of this contraction-paralysis are dosage dependent.

This response of the contraction-paralysis to scorpion venom was demonstrated in all fly larvae tested so far, such as *Calliphora, Lucilia, Musca,* and *Drosophila*, and also in larvae of *Galleria melonella* (Lepidoptera) and *Trogo-*

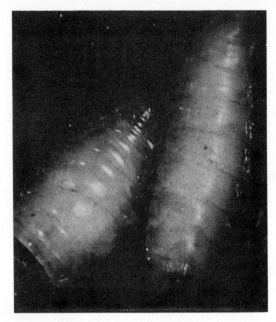

FIGURE 1.   Contraction-paralysis response of a *Sarcophaga* larva to the injection of 0.5 µg of *L. quinquestriatus* venom (left), compared with the normal appearance of a larva injected with saline (right)

derma granarium (Coleoptera).

The central nervous system of fly larvae is condensed into a mass of nerve tissue located in the thorax (Snodgrass, 1935). The abdominal part can be completely separated from the central nervous system (Fraenkel, 1935) through a ligature made beneath the thoracal region, thus losing mobility and tonus. As shown in Figure 2, injection of scorpion venom into the isolated abdomen immediately caused a contraction.

It may be assumed that the immediate and general contracture of the segmental muscles in the fly larvae when treated with scorpion venom is an additional expression of the well known peripheral excitatory effect (Zlotkin and Shulov, 1969) of scorpion venom. This assumption is strengthened by observations of the effect of scorpion venom on the ligated larvae, which do not contain the central nervous system. It is interesting that veratrine which mimics the *L. quinquestriatus* venom's direct stimulatory effect on isolated toad muscle (Adam and Weiss, 1959) imitates also its contraction-paralysis effect on fly larvae.

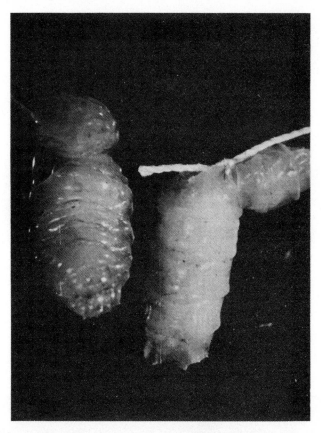

FIGURE 2.   Ligated larvae injected into the hind part: on the left with 0.5 μg of *L. quinquestriatus* venom, on the right with saline as a control

The above response of fly larvae to scorpion venom was used as a test system for its quantitative estimation. A contraction-paralysis of a minimal duration of 5 seconds was defined as a standard positive response. When graded amounts of scorpion venom are injected into groups of fly larvae a typical sigmoid dose-response curve is obtained. The amount of venom causing a positive response in 50 percent of test larvae (effective dose or ED_{50}) is defined as a unit of toxicity and called the Contraction-Paralysis Unit (CPU). For the sake of convenience and rapidity in the determination of CPU the method of estimating the fifty percent end point developed by Reed and Muench (1938) was used. The method of injection and of determination of a positive response is shown in Figures 3–6.

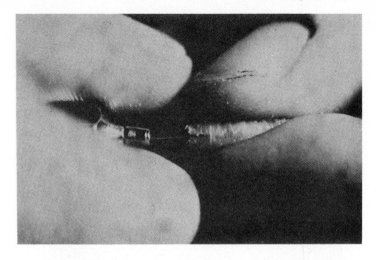

FIGURE 3.   A *Sarcophaga* larva is placed on the needle connected to a micrometrically operated syringe. The needle is inserted ventrally into the last abdominal segment

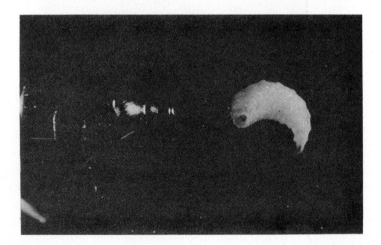

FIGURE 4.   The larva on the needle prior to injection showing active twisting movements

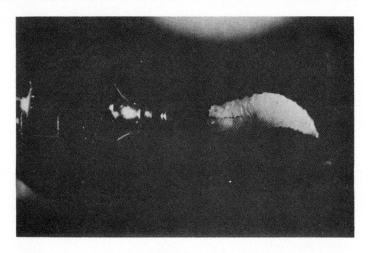

FIGURE 5.   The larva already responding while the venom solution is injected. A local contraction at the tip of the inserted needle may be seen

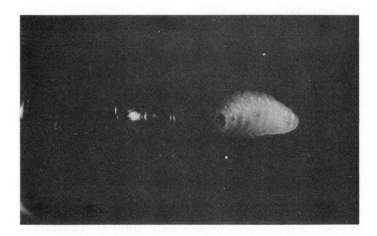

FIGURE 6.   Final contracting effect of the venom accompanied by complete immobility

TABLE 1   A comparison between the CPU and mice LD_{50} values of different scorpion venoms

Scorpion venom	$LD50[1]$ $\mu g/20$ g mouse	$CPU[2]$ $\mu g/larva$
Leiurus quinquestriatus	5.1	0.22
Androctonus aeneas aeneas[3]	6.2	0.05
Androctonus mauretanicus mauretanicus[3]	6.3	0.47
Androctonus australis	7.0	0.29
Centruroides santa maria[5]	7.7	3.82
Androctonus crassicauda[3]	8.0	0.68
Tityus serrulatus[4]	8.6	2.17
Buthiscus bicalcaratus[5]	12.0	0.07
Centruroides limpidus tecomanus[5]	13.7	0.22
Androctonus amoreuxi[3]	15.0	0.36
Buthacus leptochelis[5]	15.3	0.09
Buthus occitanus tunetanus[3]	17.9	0.05
Buthacus arenicola[5]	19.8	0.07
Buthus occitanus paris[3]	83.0	0.03
Buthotus minax[2]	85.0	0.30
Parabuthus transvaalicus[3]	85.0	0.35
Scorpio maurus[3]	Inactive[6]	Inactive[7]
Opistophtalmus glabifrons[3]	Inactive[8]	Inactive[9]

1 Estimated according to Behrens and Karber (1935).
2 Tested on *Sarcophaga* larvae.
3 Obtained from F. G. Celo, Zweibrücken (Germany).
4 Granted by Butantan Institute.
5 Granted by Prof. L. Balozet (Institut Pasteur d'Algérie)
6 Maximal dose injected 2,832 μg/mouse.
7 Maximal dose injected 15 μg/larva.
8 Maximal dose injected 430 μg/mouse.
9 Maximal dose injected 15 μg/larva.

It should be noted here that the contraction-paralysis as well as the lethal effects of scorpion venom on fly larvae can be neutralized by a scorpion antiserum.

The contraction-paralysis effect of different scorpion venoms on fly larvae was compared to their lethal effect on mice. Table 1 presents data on 18 scorpion venoms. The venoms are listed in the order of their toxicity to mice and may be divided into four groups where the LD_{50} ranges are 5—9

12–20, above 80 μg/mouse, and nontoxic. The two venoms of the latter group did not show any effect on fly larvae. But in the other 16 scorpion venoms no correlation existed between the effects on mice and fly larvae. For example, in the first group of venoms the Contraction-Paralysis Unit ranged between 0.05–3.8 μg/larva. Another example is the venom of *Buthus occitanus paris* which had only a very weak effect on mice (LD$_{50}$ 83 μg/ mouse) but was the most potent venom on fly larvae (CPU 0.03 μg/larva).

The absence of a correlation between lethal effects to mice and the larval contraction-paralysis effect of the different venoms suggests that different components in scorpion venoms are responsible for each of the two toxic activities. To check this hypothesis the venom of the North-African scorpion *Androctonus australis* was chosen as the experimental material. The toxins lethal to mice of this venom have been studied (Miranda *et al.*, 1964a, 1964b, 1966), and recently obtained as pure proteins (Rochat *et al.*, 1967). These are called toxin I (molecular weight of 6,822 and a LD$_{50}$ of 19 μg/kg) and toxin II (molecular weight of 7,249 and LD$_{50}$ of 10 μg/kg).

Solutions of pure toxins I and II were injected into *Sarcophaga* larvae in amounts ranging between 0.7 to 2.5 LD$_{50}$/20 g mouse which is equivalent to 5 to 17 μg of the crude venom. These compounds were entirely inactive on *Sarcophaga* larvae in regard to contraction-paralysis as well as lethality. As shown in Table 1, the contraction-paralysis unit of *Androctonus* venom is about 0.3 μg.

These data strongly support the hypothesis that the components of the venom effective on fly larvae are different from those toxic to mice. An attempt was then made to separate these two components by the use of starch gel electrophoresis (Figure 7).

Figure 7A represents a typical protein pattern of *Androctonus* crude venom. By testing the eluate of 40 different sections of such a run a clear separation was obtained of the fractions toxic to fly larvae and mice. Two fractions toxic to mice (labelled tx I and tx II) migrated toward the cathode but showed different mobilities. On the other hand, the material toxic to larvae appeared as a single protein band on the anode side close to the starting point. This fraction is characterized by its immediate contractive-paralyzing effect. The larvae injected with the different starch gel eluates were kept until pupation. The lethality was limited to the three sections marked by the arrows LT (Figure 7A). Therefore there was a complete correlation between the lethality and contraction-paralysis, suggesting that the same compound is responsible for both phenomena.

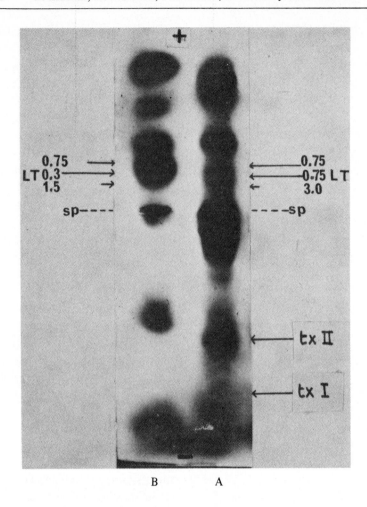

B   A

FIGURE 7.   Starch gel zone electrophoresis of the crude (A) and partially purified (B) venom of *A. australis:* A. separation of crude venom. The arrows labelled tx I and tx II indicate the location of the fractions toxic to mice corresponding to toxin I and toxin II (Rochat *et al.*, 1967); B. separation of material toxic to larvae obtained by Sephadex gel filtration (see Figure 8). Staining with amidoblack

For testing the activity the unstained gels were cut into 40 sections. The arrows (LT) point to the position of the three consecutive sections containing eluates causing contraction-paralysis and lethality to larvae. The relative toxicity of each eluate is expressed by the length of the arrow and by the number on each arrow which refers to the volume of eluate (μl) corresponding to one CPU

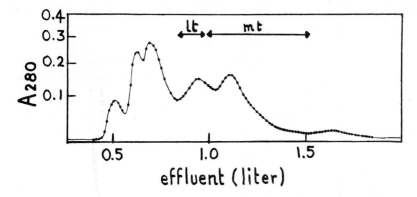

FIGURE 8.   Sephadex G-50 gel filtration of 1 g of *A. australis* venom after water extraction and dialysis. A 5 × 100 cm column was used. Eluant: 0.1 M ammonium acetate buffer, pH 8.5. The flow rate was 50 ml/hr and fractions of 15 ml were collected. lt, larvae-toxic fraction; mt, mice-toxic fraction

Figure 8 shows a Sephadex G-50 gel filtration pattern of 1 g of venom following water extraction and dialysis. The fraction toxic to mice (mt) and larvae (lt) can be also differentiated in this system. They appear in two adjacent peaks of the elution pattern indicating that the larval toxin may be of a higher molecular weight.

Figure 7B shows the electrophoretic separation of a sample of the fraction toxic to larvae previously purified by Sephadex G-50 filtration. The presence of a large number of bands indicates that it is still a mixture of proteins. The migration of the active band separated from the Sephadex-purified fraction is identical to that observed in the crude venom. Thus, the component active on larvae had been purified by Sephadex G-50 filtration and separated from the proteins toxic to mice. Its proteinic nature is suggested from its inactivation by proteolytic enzymes or the addition of antiserum to whole venom.

From the data presented in this communication it may be concluded that the toxic effects of *Androctonus australis* venom on mice and fly larvae are caused by different proteins.

The existence of distinct toxic proteins with specific effects on mammals and insects has been already demonstrated (Frontali and Grasso, 1964) in the venom of the black widow spider *Latrodectus tredecimguttatus*, using similar techniques. Different proteins causing lethality and typical envenomation symptoms on hamsters or mice, and a paralytic knock-down effect to adult flies were distinguished.

According to our present knowledge on the mode of action of scorpion venoms (Zlotkin and Shulov, 1969) the effects of the venom, both on mice or larvae, can be ascribed to a neurotoxicity of an excitatory nature. With this background the specificity of action of different components of *A. australis* venom on different organisms is surprising. This suggests an experimental approach to the problem on two main lines, one to compare the molecular structure of these discrete toxic proteins, and the other to specify their mode of action at the neurophysiological level.

SUMMARY

Injection of scorpion venom into intact or ligated (thus nullifying the central nervous system) larvae of blowflies causes an immediate paralysis accompanied by strong contraction of the test animals, demonstrating the peripheral nerve-muscle stimulating effect of the venom. The duration of this contractive paralysis may range from several seconds to several hours, depending on the amount of venom injected. This effect of scorpion venom on fly larvae formed the basis of a very rapid and sensitive test for the quantitative estimation of scorpion venom.

The venom of eighteen different species of scorpions was tested for its contractive-paralyzing activity in fly larvae and its lethal effect on mice (LD_{50} estimations). No correlation was found between the two biological activities. These data suggested the possibility that there are different components of scorpion venom responsible for each of the above two biological activities. This hypothesis was verified by the following experimental results:

Purified proteins from *Androctonus australis* venom which were highly toxic to mice were completely ineffective against fly larvae when tested for their contractive-paralyzing activity. Furthermore these proteins were not lethal to the larvae.

A clear separation between larvae and mice toxic components was achieved both by starch gel electrophoresis and Sephadex-G-50 column chromatography of the crude venom of *A. australis*. It has been shown that the contractive paralyzing fraction was the sole fraction lethal to fly larvae. An electrophoretical analysis of the Sephadex larval-active fraction revealed the presence of several protein bands, only one of which contained the larval toxic activity. In its mobility characteristics the above component closely resembled those of the larvae-active component previously separated by an identical procedure from the crude venom. The above mentioned larvae-active component was ineffective on mice.

It is concluded that scorpion venoms may contain different components with specific toxic effects against different groups of animals.

References

Adam, K. R. and C. Weiss 1959 'Actions of scorpion venom on skeletal muscle.' *Brit. J. Pharmacol.*, 14: 334–339.

Bearg, W. J. 1961 'Scorpions: Biology and effect of their venom.' *Agric. Exptl. Stat. Univ. Arkansas Bull.* 649: 1–34.

Behrens, B. and C. Karber 1935 'Wie sind Reihenwersuche für biologische Auswertungen am zweckmässigsten anzuordnen?' *Arch. Exp. Pathol. Pharmakol.*, 177: 379–388.

Fraenkel, G. 1935 'A hormone causing pupation in the blowfly *Calliphora erythrocephala*.' *Proc. Roy. Soc. (B)*, 118: 1–5.

Frontali, N. and A. Grasso 1964 'Separation of three toxicologically different protein components from the venom of the spider *Latrodectus tredecimguttatus*.' *Arch. Biochem. Biophys.*, 106: 213–218.

Gomez, M. V. and C. R. Diniz 1966 'Separation of toxic components from the Brazilian scorpion *Tityus serrulatus* venom.' *Mem. Inst. Butantan Simp. Internac.*, 33: 899–902.

Lissitzky, S., F. Miranda, P. Etzensperger and J. Mercier 1956 'Sur la toxicité du venin de deux espèces de Scorpions nord-africains.' *Compt. Rend. Soc. Biol.*, 150: 741–743.

Miranda, F. 1964 'Purification et Caractérisation des Neurotoxines des Venins de Scorpions (Scorpamines).' Doctorat d'etat es-Sciences Physiques, Marseille.

Miranda, F., H. Rochat and S. Lissitzky 1964a 'Sur les neurtoxines de deux espèces de scorpions nord-africains I. Purification des neurotoxines (scorpamines) d'*Androctonus australis* (L.) et de *Buthus occitanus* (Am.).' *Toxicon*, 2: 51–69.

Miranda. F., H. Rochat and S. Lissitzky 1964b 'Sur les neurotoxines de deux espèces de scorpions nord-africains. III. Déterminations préliminaires aux études de structure sur les neurotoxines (scorpamines) d'*Androctonus australis* et de *Buthus occitanus* (Am.).' *Toxicon*, 2: 123–138.

Miranda, F., H. Rochat, C. Rochat and S. Lissitzky, 1966 'Complexes moléculaires présentés par les neurotoxines animales. I. Neurotoxines de venins de scorpions *Androctonus australis* (L.) et *Buthus occitanus* (Am.).' *Toxicon*, 4: 123–144.

Reed, L. J. and H. Muench 1938 'A simple method of estimating fifty per cent end points.' *Amer. J. Hyg.*, 27: 493–497.

Rochat, H. 1964 'Contribution à l'Identification de Diverses Formes Actives des Neurotoxines des Scorpions.' Doctorat d'Etat en Pharmacie, Marseille.

Rochat, C., H. Rochat, F. Miranda and S. Lissitzky 1967 'Purification and some properties of the neurotoxins of *Androctonus australis Hector*.' *Biochemistry*, 6: 578–585.

Snodgrass, E. E. 1935 *'Principles of Insect Morphology*.' McGraw Hill Publ.

Watt, D. D. 1964 'Biochemical studies of the venom from the scorpion *Centruroides sculpturatus*.' *Toxicon*, 2: 171–180.

Zlotkin, E. and A. Shulov 1969 'Recent studies on the mode of action of scorpion neurotoxins. A review.' *Toxicon*, 7: 217–221.

EFFECT OF SCORPION VENOM *CENTRUROIDES SCULPTURATUS* ON THE CAROTID BODY AND SUPERIOR CERVICAL GANGLION OF THE CAT

R. A. PATTERSON

Department of Zoology, Arizona State Univeristy, Tempe, Arizona, U.S.A.

and

D. WOOLEY

Barrow Neurological Institute, Phoenix, Arizona, U.S.A.

INTRODUCTION

AN ADVANTAGE of studying scorpion venoms is that they tend to induce unusual responses when tested on practically any irritable tissue. Only vertebrate nerve trunks appear unresponsive—presumably a result of the protective lipoid material which surrounds them. Scorpion venoms seem to affect pharmacologically exposed areas of nerve and muscle. Primarily, effects of various scorpion venoms have been investigated with respect to neurons, myo-neural junctions, and both smooth and skeletal muscle. Results as Zlotkin and Shulov (1969) point out suggest that these venoms—at least those that have been studied in depth—influence ion movement during and after the action potential. Also, venoms appear to enhance release of acetylcholine at vertebrate myo-neural junctions. They also act directly on both skeletal and smooth muscle, even in the presence of competitive blocking agents of acetylcholine. While it is unlikely that every scorpion venom exhibits these actions, the actions serve as a model for describing and comparing effects of other scorpion venoms. In this presentation we shall point out other sites which are affected by venom of a scorpion from the southwestern United Stated and northern Mexico, *Centruroides sculpturatus.*

This investigation stemmed from earlier work carried out (Patterson, 1962) to characterize the action of this venom on several different types of smooth muscle. We concluded that this venom caused post-synaptic activation of the visceral parasympathetic nervous network. Incidentally, in the intact anesthetized animal, venom causes inhibition of visceral smooth muscle activity (Patterson, 1960), an effect either of the sympathetic control of intestinal smooth muscle or the releases of epinephrine from the adrenal medulla. However, in isolated smooth muscle, *in vitro*, this venom stimulates smooth muscle in a complex manner (Patterson, 1962). Atropine which blocks muscle stimulating effects of acetylcholine prevents some, but not all, of the action of this venom on the guinea pig ileum. This suggests that venom acts directly on smooth muscle as well as through the effector neurons of the parasympathetic nervous system. The direct effect on this muscle was not blocked by antihistmaines. Hexamethonium which blocks ganglionic stimulation by nicotine did not prevent the venom induced response.

We extended this study to examine the action of venom on the superior cervical ganglion of the cat to characterize, if possible, the effect of venom on another cholinergic system. Post-ganglionic fibers of this structure innervate, among other structures, the nictitating membrane. The effector neurons function adrenergically. The ganglion is primarily cholinergic, although some chromaffin tissue is present producing catecholamines of unknown function. It has been suggested by Eccles and Libet (1961) that nor-epinephrine may have a hyper-polarizing effect on the post-synaptic sites. We hoped to determine whether venom caused contraction of the membrane by ganglionic activation directly or indirectly as a result of general sympathetic activity. We assumed that since no epinephrine-like effect had been detected on smooth muscle, *in vitro*, the venom would not effect the membrane. Later we discovered that this structure will respond to exogenous acetylcholine as noted by Florey (1962).

METHODS

The technique used was described by Trendelenberg (1959). In the nembutalized cat, an ascending sympathetic nerve was teased free from the vagal trunk in the neck and cut centrally. Electrical stimulation was applied to verify the function of these nerves both before and after separation. Response of the nictitating membrane as well as arterial pressure, ventilatory activity, and cardiac electrical activity were recorded oscillographically. The head was held rigid in a head holder. A lingual artery was cleared and cannulated for injection of test materials. A portion of the external carotid artery was cleared so that it could be clamped to prevent material injected through the artery from passing toward the eye. Instead, the injected material would pass from the occipital artery to the superior cervical ganglion through small connecting arteries. Without the clamp, the injected material would pass through the external carotid and not immediately reach the superior cervical ganglion.

In some experiments both ganglia and lingual arteries were prepared in this manner. One side of such bilateral preparations was used as a control, the other as a test site. Two types of test site preparations were used. In one set of experiments one ganglion of each cat was destroyed by crushing. In another set the ganglion was inactivated by lingual arterial injections of nicotine. Electrical stimulation of the preganglionic fibers verified the extent of inactivation and destruction.

RESULTS AND DISCUSSION

In a preliminary series cats were injected with venom both toward the ganglion and toward the eye. In all 12 animals tested with injections of venom directed toward the ganglion, the nictitating membrane responded. Doses of venom ranged from 1.0 to 0.1 mg. Nine cats injected with venom toward the eye yielded indecisive results. About half of them exhibited membrane contractions; the other half did not. In general the uninjected side which received no venom directly did not respond immediately to the venom. Two of the 13 cats did respond to some extent; 10 did not and one responded questionably. Possibly the nictitating membrane reacted as blood containing the venom recirculated to its site.

In the bilaterally prepared cats, venom was injected simultaneously through both lingual arteries toward the ganglion. In one series of 5 cats, one ganglion of each was inactivated physically by crushing; in the other series of 6 cats the ganglion of each was inactivated by nicotine. Following injection of venom, one of the 5 cats with crushed ganglia responded to venom; the other 4 did not. Venom caused contractions of the nictitating membrane in 4 of the

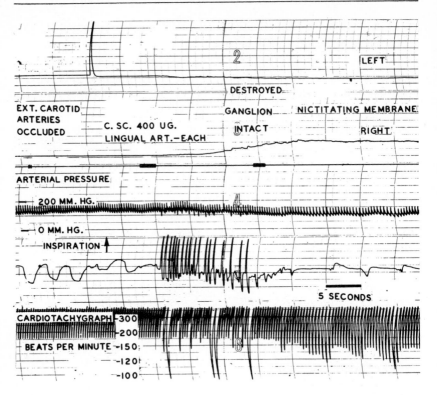

FIGURE 1.   The action of scorpion venom on a bilaterally prepared cat. Venom was injected through each lingual artery simultaneously. The left ganglion had been destroyed previously by crushing

6 nicotine-treated cats. On the control side one cat in each series failed to exhibit ganglionic stimulation following venom injection. Since nicotine inactivates the cholinoceptive sites of the post-synaptic membrane (Paton and Perry, 1957), we concluded that this venom has the capability of stimulating non-cholinergically the post synaptic membrane. Substances which activate the nicotine blocked ganglion are termed by Trendelenberg (1959) as 'non-nicotinic ganglion stimulating substances'. Evidently this scorpion venom possesses such a capability.

One other observation is apparent. In contrast to the immediate response evoked by ganglionic injection of acetylcholine and KCl, venom produced a delayed response (Figure 1). We are unable to account for this. Probably some indirect mechanism of activation is involved.

During these experiments we noted a rather severe and immediate response of the ventilatory system and a somewhat less striking effect on heart rate and arterial pressure (Figure 1). We became concerned with the cause of these effects since venom dosages were considerably below a level of 0.5 mg per kg which is required to produce immediate cardiovascular and ventilatory disturbances.

There was either no cardiac response, or there were symptoms of tachycardia, or bradycardia. In general they were transitory. When the heart slowed, blood pressure fell; when the heart accelerated, arterial pressure rose. Ventilatory responses, as seen in Figure 1, were prompt and dramatic. Either inspiratory or expiratory apnea or pronounced hyperventilation developed. Irregular breathing followed this initial phase. These effects were more common when the external carotid was clamped than when it was not clamped. Since we attempted to place the lingual cannula tip just above the bifurcation of the external and occipital arteries, we felt that venom might be stimulating the sensory regions of this area inducing ventilatory and cardiovascular responses. Stretch receptors which comprise part of the arterial pressoreceptive system are found in the enlarged bulge at the base of the occipital artery in the cat. The chemoreceptive carotid body is embedded in this structure as well. To examine this possibility we prepared cats with unilateral exposures of this region. Through a lingual artery venom was injected while the external carotid was occluded. Recordings from silver chlorided hook electrodes of nerve activity of a centrally transected branch of the IX cranial nerve which leads to this region—the carotid sinus nerve—were obtained and displayed on a Tektronix 564 oscilloscope equipped with a 2A 61 preamplifier. The preamplifier output was monitored both audially and on a conventional audio tape recorder. After preliminary work on several cats, results were obtained from 3 animals. As Figure 2 shows, nerve activity in the sinus nerve during the control exposure shows the pulsatile pressoreceptor activity associated with the cardiac cycle. After venom treatment, neural activity increased impressively. We found this response both immediately after envenomation and periodically afterwards. Since there was no elevation in the arterial pressure when venom was injected intra-lingually (in the particular test animal) we assume that the nerve activity originated in the chemoreptors of the carotid body. A cat injected with venom intravenously showed similar activity. As the condition of the animal deteriorated following envenomation, we could find repetitive responses apparently of single neurons which persisted for many seconds at a frequency of about 200 times per second. These

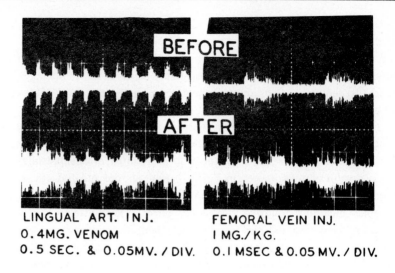

LINGUAL ART. INJ.   FEMORAL VEIN INJ.
0.4MG. VENOM   I MG./ KG.
0.5 SEC. & 0.05MV. / DIV.   0.I MSEC & 0.05 MV. / DIV.

FIGURE 2.   The effect on nerve activity in the carotid sinus nerve of venom injected through the lingual artery in one cat and through the femoral vein in another

produced distinctive buzzing sounds through the audio monitor.

While we have not yet examined the pharmacological properties of this response, Eyzaguirre (1969) has emphasized the cholinergic involvement in the chemoreceptor function of the carotid body. Since this scorpion venom is known to effect other cholinergic mechanisms, it seems likely to affect the cholinergic mechanism of this sensory system as well.

In conclusion, we would like to stress that while venom acts on cholinergic systems of the myoneural junction other portions of the nervous system respond also. In this study we found that the venom from scorpion *Centruroides sculpturatus* activates the nictitating membrane, the superior cervical ganglion and the carotid body-sinus sensory structures. All these, with the exception of the sinus stretch receptors, contain cholinergic mechanisms. It seems possible that the marked ventilatory dysfunction which occurs following scorpion envenomation may involve impaired sensory function.

SUMMARY

Effects of venom from the scorpion, *Centruroides sculpturatus*, on the superior cervical ganglion and carotid body chemoreceptor function have been studied *in situ*. Venom was injected into anesthetized cats through the lingual artery in such a manner that it passed either directly through the external carotid artery to the nictitating membrane or into the carotid body and superior cervical ganglion circulation. In the former case, venom did not enter the circulatory pathway of either the ganglion or carotid body; in the latter case venom entered the circulatory pathway of the carotid body and ganglion only. Responses were noted in recordings of tension of the nictitating membrane and of action potentials picked up from sleeve electrodes placed on the carotid body nerve.

The nictitating membrane contracted when venom passed directly to it and when venom circulated through the superior cervical ganglion without entering the circulatory pathway to the nictitating membrane. Blocking the ganglion with nicotine did not abolish the stimulating action of the venom. Venom enhanced the frequency of action potentials appearing in the carotid body nerve. This response may be related to the respiratory distress which accompanies the intra-venous administration of venom.

References

Eccles, R. M. and B. Libet 1961 'Origin and blockade of the synaptic responses of curarized sympathetic ganglia.' *J. Physiol.*, 157: 484–503.

Eyzaguirre, C. 1969 *'Physiology of the Nervous System.'* Year Book Medical Publishers Inc., Chicago, Ill.

Florey, E. 1962 'Recent studies on synaptic transmitters.' *Am. Zool.*, 2: 45–54.

Paton, W. D. M. and W. L. Perry 1953 'The relationship between depolarization and block in the cat's superior cervical ganglion.' *J. Physiol.*, 119: 43–57.

Patterson, R. A. 1960 'Physiological actions of scorpion venom.' *Am. J. Trop. Med. Hyg.*, 9: 410–414.

Patterson, R. A. 1962 'Pharmacologic action of scorpion venom on intestinal smooth muscle.' *Toxic Appl. Pharmacol.*, 4: 710–719.

Trendelenburg, U. 1959 'Non-nicotinic ganglion stimulating substances.' *Fed. Proc.*, 18: 1001–1005.

Zlotkin, E. and A. S. Shulov 1969 'Recent studies on the mode of action of scorpion neurotoxins.' *Toxicon*, 7: 217–221.

PURIFICATION AND MODE OF ACTION OF TOXIN FROM *ELEDONE CIRROSA*

N. M. McDONALD and G. A. COTTRELL

Wellcome Laboratories of Pharmacology, Gatty Marine Laboratory,
University of St. Andrews, Fife, Scotland

INTRODUCTION

PREVIOUS WORK has shown that the venom-secreting posterior salivary glands of many cephalopod molluscs, particularly the octopods, contain a toxin that causes a flaccid paralysis when injected into decapod crustaceans. An exactly similar paralysis is observed in naturally envenomated crustaceans. The toxic factor was shown to be a macromolecule in several species of cephalopods by Livon and Briot (1906) and Ghiretti (1959, 1960). Ghiretti was able to isolate a toxic protein from the posterior salivary glands of two species of *Octopus* and one species of *Sepia*. The protein, which he named 'cephalotoxin', was also shown to be present in *Octopus* saliva.

The subject of this report is the toxin of *Eledone cirrosa* (Octopoda, Cephalopoda) (see Figure 1). The toxin has been extracted, and partially purified, from the posterior salivary glands. Some of the biochemical and pharmacological properties of the toxin are described (Table 1). It shows some similarity to 'cephalotoxin.'

MATERIALS AND METHODS

Specimens of *Eledone cirrosa* and the Norwegian lobster *Nephrops norvegicus* were obtained from local fishermen. Specimens of the shore crab *Carcinus maenas* were collected from local beaches. The animals were kept in large tanks of fresh, aerated sea water until required.

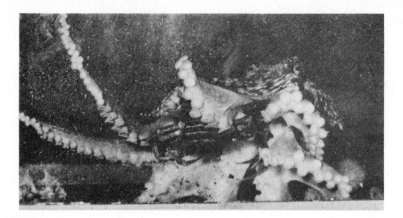

FIGURE   1.   A specimen of *Eledone cirrosa* attacking a specimen of the crab *Carcinus maenas*

TABLE 1   Biochemical tests performed on crude extracts of toxin from the posterior salivary glands of *Eledone cirrosa*

Test	Result of Assay	Conclusion
Crude extract heated to 100° C for 10 min cooled and assayed	Negative	Toxin is heat-labile
Crude extract dialyzed against cold dilute saline and assayed	Positive	Toxin is non-dialyzable
Crude extract treated with 10% TCA. Precipitate centrifuged down. Supernatant neutralised and assayed.	Negative	Toxin precipitated
pH of crude extract adjusted to 4. Precipitate centrifuged down. Supernatant neutralised and assayed	Negative	Toxin precipitated

Extraction procedure
The posterior salivary glands were removed from specimens of *Eledone* that had first been killed by rapid destruction of the brain with sharp scissors.

The glands were either used immediately or stored frozen at $-12°$ C.

To extract the toxin, the glands were homogenized in cold 2.5% NaCl, in a pre-cooled glass homogenizer (final volume 10 ml of saline/g of gland). The homogenate was stirred automatically for 4–5 hr in a cold room, then centrifuged at 25,000 g for 20 min at $1°$ C. The supernatant, a semi-opaque liquid with a pH of 6.2–6.4, contained the toxic activity and was called the crude extract. The precipitate could be re-extracted as before, but as it did not add significantly to the activity it was generally discarded.

Bioassay

Crude and purified extracts of the toxin were assayed on *Carcinus*. If crabs were in short supply, specimens of *Nephrops* were used instead. Both species showed a similar susceptibility to the toxin. Crude and purified extracts were systematically diluted and injected in 0.8 ml aliquots into groups of 4–5 assay animals, kept in bowls of aerated sea water. Mortality was noted at 48 hr. All the extracts assayed were approximately isotonic with crustacean hemolymph. The results were calculated according to the method of Reed and Meunch (1938). A 'crab unit' was defined as the amount of toxin present in one dose of the particular dilution of extract required to paralyze half the assay animals in one group in 48 hr.

Protein estimation

Protein was estimated throughout according to the method of Lowry *et al.* (1951). Bovine serum albumin was used as a standard.

Ammonium sulphate fractionation

Cold saturated ammonium sulphate solution was added dropwise, with constant agitation, to crude extracts (pH 6.2–6.4, protein content approximately 10 mg/ml) until the desired degree of saturation was reached. The resulting mixture was allowed to stand at $1°$ C for at least 30 min when any precipitate was centrifuged down at 3000 g for 20 min at $1°$ C. The supernatant was kept for further fractionation and the precipitate redissolved in distilled water, dialyzed against cold dilute saline to remove excess ammonium sulphate, and assayed for toxic activity.

Molecular sieve chromatography

In an attempt to purify the toxin further, crude and ammonium sulphate-purified extracts were chromatographed on columns containing either

Sephadex G-75 or G-200 in 0.9% NaCl solution. Fractions were collected automatically and monitored for protein by measuring their optical density of 280 mμ. The contents of tubes corresponding to individual protein peaks were pooled, freeze-dried and assayed for toxic activity.

Starch gel electrophoresis

To determine the degree of heterogeneity of crude and purified extracts of toxin, electrophoresis was performed on horizontal starch gel blocks in 0.2 M borate buffer at pH 8.4. Samples were generally concentrated beforehand by freeze-drying and applied to vertical cuts made in the gels on pieces of Whatman No. 1 filter paper. After 6—16 hr (10 v/cm), electrophoresis was terminated and the gels were sliced in two, longitudinally and parallel to the flat surface. They were then stained for 30 min in a saturated solution of Amidoschwarz 10B dye in methanol/glacial acetic acid/water (5:1:5 by volume). The gels were then destained on the apparatus of Stanton (1965) and stored in the same solution used to dissolve the dye.

Pharmacology of toxic extracts

Preliminary experiments were made on nerve-muscle systems in the abdomen of *Nephrops* to determine the mode of action of the toxin. Three preparations were used: (1) The deep extensor muscles and the nerve supplying them. The action of snake, spider and scorpion venoms on the same preparation in crayfish was studied by Parnas and Russell (1967). The system in *Nephrops* is essentially similar to that studied in the crayfish and lobster (Abbott and Parnas, 1965; Parnas and Attwood, 1966). The preparation was pinned in a small bath containing crustacean saline (Attwood, 1963). Twitch contractions were observed when the nerve to the muscles was stimulated with 2–3 sec burst of 1 msec pulses delivered at 50 Hz. To test the effect of the toxin, the bath solution was replaced by crude extracts, previously dialyzed against crustacean saline. The nerve to the muscle was stimulated every 5 min as before and the mechanical response of the muscles was observed. (2) Similar experiments were made on the superficial flexor muscles. The same preparation in crayfish was used to study the action of *Condylactis* toxin (Shapiro, 1968). As in the crayfish (Kennedy and Takeda, 1965) the superficial flexors of *Nephrops* are a thin ventral sheet of muscle fibres supplied by a posterior branch of the third root to the abdominal ganglia. In this study the muscles were isolated, together with the nerve supplying them, and a portion of the ventral nerve cord. The preparation was pinned in a small bath containing crustacean saline. The procedure outlined above for testing the response of the deep extensor muscles to indirect stimulation was repeated. In addition, spontaneous activity in the nerve supplying the muscles could be monitored by raising it out of the saline onto a pair of platinum recording electrodes, connected through a differential amplifier to an oscilloscope. Finally, the electrical responses of the muscles to spontaneous and induced nerve impulses were recorded intracellularly with glass microelectrodes, filled with 3M KCl, connected through a negative-capacitance preamplifier to an osscilloscope. These responses were observed after exposure of the preparation to dialyzed toxic extracts as outlined above. (3) Another preparation was the dorsal muscle receptor organ. The pharmacology of the same preparation in crayfish was first studied by Wiersma , *et al* (1953). The receptor organ was exposed by removing the deep extensor muscle preparation described above. The nerve supplying the organ was carefully dissected free of its other branches, and was raised out of the saline on a pair of recording electrodes to record the tonic output of the slowly-adapting receptor organ. The bath solution was replaced by dialyzed crude extracts of toxin, and the output of the receptor organ monitored at regular (10 min) intervals.

RESULTS

Ammonium sulphate fractionation

The toxin was precipitated from the crude extract at 67% ammonium sulphate saturation. A minimum of 75% of the toxic activity was recovered and about a two-fold purification was achieved (Table 2).

Molecule sieve chromatography

Chromatography of crude extracts of toxin on Sephadex G-200 showed that the toxin was retarded, emerging in a distinct peak between two other peaks corresponding to the void column and the total column volume (Figure 2). When crude extracts were chromatographed on G-75 columns, two large peaks were obtained and the toxic activity was found in the first, corresponding to the void volume (Figure 3). The toxin was therefore excluded from the gel. Prior precipitation of the toxin, however, altered its behaviour on Sephadex columns. Ammonium sulphate-purified extracts chromatographed on G-75 columns gave five peaks and the toxin was retarded by the gel, emerging in a smaller peak, after the void volume (Figure 4). This toxic

TABLE 2   Purification of toxin from the posterior salivary glands of *Eledone cirrosa*

Stages of Purification	Protein Concn. (mg/ml)	Activity (crab units/ml)	Specific Activity
1. Extraction with 2.5% NaCl solution	9.2	15	1.6
2. Precipitation with ammonium sulphate solution, 0–67% saturation	4.1	12	2.9
3. Molecular sieve chromatography on Sephadex G-75 in 0.9% NaCl	1.23	6	4.9

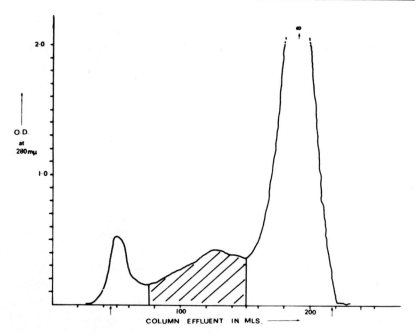

FIGURE 2.   Chromatography of crude extract of *Eledone* toxin on Sephadex G-200 in a 0.9% NaCl solution.
The two arrows indicate the void volume and the total column volume respectively. The cross hatched area shows where the toxic activity was found

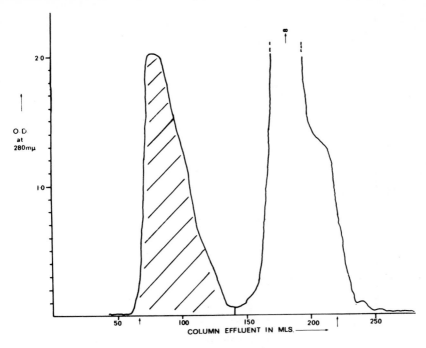

FIGURE 3.   Chromatography of crude extract of *Eledone* toxin on Sephadex G-75 in 0.9% NaCl solution.
Symbols as for Figure 2

fraction from the G-75 column was called the Sephadex-purified extract and has not yet been purified further. Typical figures for the purification are given in Tabe 2. It will be seen that a threefold purification was achieved. LD_{50} values of 5−10 mg of toxin protein/kg of crab were obtained for the Sephadex-purified extract.

Starch gel electrophoresis

When crude extracts were subjected to starch gel electrophoresis, a number of bands were observed, some migrating to the anode and others migrating to the cathode. When the Sephadex-purified extract was electrophoresed, the number of visible bands was reduced to two, and both moved towards the cathode. Both these bands corresponded to bands found in the crude extract, as was demonstrated by running both crude and Sephadex-purified extracts on one gel, when like bands joined up to form one continuous band (Figure 5).

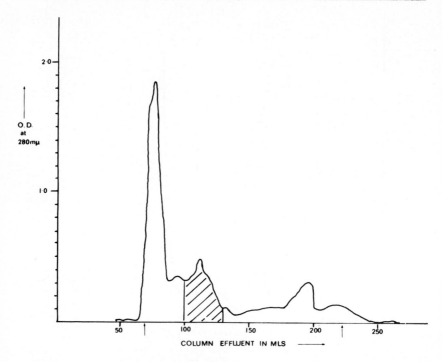

FIGURE 4.   Chromatography of ammonium sulphate-purified extract of *Eledone* toxin on Sephadex G-75 in 0.9 NaCl solution.
    Symbols as for Figure 2

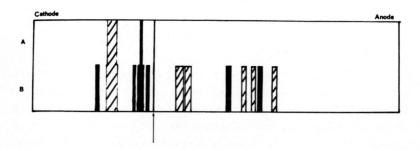

FIGURE 5.   Diagram of a starch gel electrophorerogram comparing A) a Sephadex-purified extract, with B) a crude extract, of *Eledone* toxin. Borate buffer pH 8.4 Running time 10 hr at 200 v. Arrow indicates the origin

Pharmacology of toxic extracts

The results of the preliminary experiments showed that dialyzed crude extracts of toxin blocked the mechanical responses of both the deep extensor muscles and superficial flexor muscles to stimulation through their respective nerves. A toxic extract containing 1 mg protein/ml was sufficient to cause a complete block in both preparations in 30—35 min. Even undiluted dialyzed crude extract took 20 min to effect a complete block. Ammonium sulphate-purified extracts containing 1 mg protein/ml blocked the superficial flexor muscle preparation in a similar time. The block was not reversed by washing.

Experiments where superficial flexor muscle fibres were impaled with microelectrodes showed that both spontaneous and indirectly induced junctional potentials were reduced in amplitude and finally abolished 35 min after exposure of the preparation to ammonium sulphate-purified extracts of toxin (1 mg protein/ml). Control experiments with boiled extracts (see Table 1) showed that they blocked neither the electrical nor the mechanical response of the muscles to stimulation of their nerves. Typical spontaneous activity could still be recorded from the nerve innervating the superficial flexor muscles in blocked preparations, indicating that nerve conduction was not affected.

The tonic output of the slowly-adapting muscle receptor organ was not affected by exposure to undiluted dialyzed crude extracts of toxin, indicating again that nerve conduction was not affected.

DISCUSSION

Eledone toxin is a macromolecule which seems to behave in all respects as a typical protein. The behaviour of the toxin on Sephadex columns is interesting. Results showed that when crude extracts are chromatographed the toxin was excluded from G-75 columns and retarded by G-200 columns. Thus a M.W. in the range 70,000—700,000 (exclusion limits for G-75 and G-200 respectively) was suggested. However, after prior precipitation with ammonium sulphate solution, the toxin was retarded on G-75 columns, which suggested a M.W. of under 70,000. The behaviour of the toxin on Sephadex columns could be explained by supposing that it occurs in the crude extract associated with a larger molecule, the complex being dissociated in the presence of high concentrations of ammonium sulphate. Neurotoxins from other species are well-known for their ability to complex with other proteins

(Miranda *et al.*, 1964; Meldrum, 1965). The Sephadex-purified extract was not homogeneous, as was shown by starch gel electrophoresis at pH 8.4. The two visible bands moved towards the cathode, indicating isoelectric points above pH 8.4. It is possible that a single band represented two or more separate proteins with identical electrophoretic behaviour. But since it seems probable that one or both of the bands observed contained the toxic activity, it is tentatively proposed that *Eledone* toxin is a basic protein(s) with a M.W. of less than 70,000.

Eledone toxin shows obvious similarities to 'cephalotoxin.' Both are protein toxins isolated from the posterior salivary glands of venomous cephalopods which cause a flaccid paralysis when injected into decapod crustaceans. 'Cephalotoxin' gave four bands on starch gel electrophorerograms at pH 8.5, but the number of bands was reduced to three after adsorption of the protein on calcium phosphate gels. Sephadex-purified extracts of *Eledone* toxin gave two visible bands on starch gel electrophorerograms at pH 8.4; both also migrated to the cathode. Many neurotoxins from different phyla have now been highly purified. They show remarkable similarities of structure, the great majority being small basic proteins or polypeptides (Miranda *et al.*, 1964). Although *Eledone* toxin has only been partially purified its structure seems to conform to the general pattern observed in other neurotoxins.

The primary site of action of many venoms seems to be at the level of the neuromuscular transmission (Russell, 1967). Effects on nervous transmission are less often observed, though this may be due to the relative inability of the toxins to penetrate the axonal sheath. The preliminary results obtained with crude and partially purified extracts of *Eledone* toxin showed that it blocked indirectly induced muscle contractions but did not affect nervous transmission when tested on nerve-muscle preparations in the abdomen of *Nephrops*. Thus the mode of action of *Eledone* toxin, as it has so far been elucidated, seems similar to that of other venom toxins.

Further studies are in progress to establish more precisely the site of action of the toxin.

ACKNOWLEDGMENTS

We wish to thank Mr. J. Brown for collecting the crabs, unfailingly and in all weathers. We are also very grateful to Mr. M. G. Stanton for his invaluable advice and assistance. One of us (N.M. McD.) acknowledges the award of a Wellcome Research Travel Grant to attend the Symposium.

SUMMARY

A toxin was extracted from the posterior salivary glands of *Eledone cirrosa*, and partially purified by ammonium sulphate fractionation and molecular sieve chromatography on Sephadex. The partially purified toxin is a basic protein(s) with a M.W, of less than 70,000. Preliminary experiments, made on nerve-muscle preparations in the abdomen of *Nephrops*, showed that crude and ammonium sulphate-purified extracts of toxin blocked the electrical and mechanical responses of muscles to stimulation through their nerves, but did not seem to affect nervous transmission.

References

Abbott, B. C. and I. Parnas 1965 'Electrical and mechanical responses in deep abdominal extensor muscles of the crayfish and lobster.' *J. Gen. Physiol.*, 48: 919–931.

Attwood, H. L. 1963 'Muscle fibre properties in fast and slow contractions in *Carcinus.*' *Comp. Biochem. Physiol.*, 10: 77–81.

Ghiretti, F. 1959 'Cephalotoxin: the crab paralyzing agent of the posterior salivary glands of cephalopods.' *Nature*, 183: 1192–1193.

Ghiretti, F. 1960 'Toxicity of *Octopus* saliva against Crustacea.' *Ann. N.Y. Acad. Sci.*, 90: 726–741.

Kennedy, D. and K. Takeda 1965 'Reflex control of abdominal flexor muscles in the crayfish. II. The tonic system.' *J. Exp. Biol.*, 43: 229–246.

Livon, C. et A. Briot 1906 'Sur le suc salivaire des Cephalopodes.' *J. Physiol. Pathol. Gen.*, 8: 1–9.

Lowry, O. H., N. J. Roseborough, A. L. Farr and R. J. Randall 1951 'Protein measurement with the Folin phenol reagent.' *J. Biol. Chem.*, 193: 265–275.

Meldrum, B. S. 1965 'The action of snake venoms on nerve and muscle. The pharmacology of phospholipase A and polypeptide toxins.' *Pharmacol. Rev.*, 17: 393–445.

Miranda, F., H. Rochat et S. Lissitsky 1964 'Sur les neurotoxines de deux especes de scorpions Nord-Africains. II. Proprietes des neurotoxines (scorpamines) d'*Androctonus australis* (L.) et de *Buthus occitanus* (Am.).' *Toxicon*, 2: 113–138.

Parnas, I. and H. L. Attwood 1966 'Phasic and tonic neuromuscular systems in the abdominal extensor muscles of the crayfish and rock lobster.' *Comp. Biochem. Physiol.*, 18: 701–723

Parnas, I. and F. E. Russell 1967 'Effects of venoms on nerve, muscle and neuromuscular junction.' In: Russell, F. E. and P. R. Saunders, (eds), *Animal Toxins*. pp. 401–415. Pergamon Press, New York.

Reed, L. J. and H. Meunch 1938 'A simple method for fifty per cent end points.' *Am. J. Hyg.*, 27: 493–497.

Russell, F. E. 1967 'Pharmacology of animal venoms.' *Clin. Pharmacol. Ther.*, 8: 849–873.

Stanton, M. G. 1965 'Rapid removal of background dye from zone electrophorerograms.' *Anal. Biochem.*, 12: 310–315.

Shapiro, B. I. 1968 'A site of action of toxin from the anemone *Condylactis gigantea*.' *Comp. Biochem. Physiol.*, 27: 519–531.

Wiersma, C. A. G., E. Furshpan and E. Florey 1953 'Physiological and pharmacological observations on muscle receptor organs of the crayfish, *Cambarus clarkii*, Girard.' *J. Exp. Biol.*, 30: 136–150.

THE ACTION OF THE TOXINS FROM
GYMNODINIUM BREVE

B. C. ABBOTT and Z. PASTER

Department of Biological Sciences,
University of Southern California, University Park, Los Angeles, California,
U.S.A.

THE ASSOCIATION of *Gymnodinium breve* (dinoflagellate) with the 'red tide' and mass mortalities of marine animals along the southeast coasts of the United States and the Gulf of Mexico is well documented (Wilson and Ray, 1956; McFarren *et al.*, 1965; Ray and Aldrich, 1965). There have been several studies concerned with the toxicity of *G. breve* cells as well as with the chemical properties of its toxin (Cummins *et al.*, 1967; Spikes *et al.*, 1968; Martin and Chatterjee, 1969).

In nature *G. breve* blooms periodically during the year, but laboratory blooms have been elusive. In some laboratories it has taken 16 months from original inoculation until an adequate harvest was available (Spikes *et al.*, 1968) with a maximum of cells at $22.4 \times 10^6/1$.

The purpose of this paper is to show that mass cultures after a short period of growth are feasible under laboratory conditions, and that these cultures contain at least two kinds of biologically active toxins.

G. breve cultures are characterized by an extremely long lag period, 6–10 days after inoculation, and a mean generation time of 6.6 days. In our experiments a synthetic medium was used composed of inorganic salts and three vitamins, namely; biotin 0.5 μg/1, thiamine 1 mg/l and B_{12} 1 μg/l. In order to support a good growth of this organism with a population of $30–40 \times 10^6$ cells/1 in 30 days, it was necessary to inoculate at least 3000 cells/ml. The total number of cells can be doubled by adding Gibberellic acid (G.A.) to the growth medium. A concentration of 10^{-7}M G. A. can promote optimal growth of *G. breve*, while higher concentrations, above 5×10^{-7}M were inhibitory.

The growth curves of *G. breve* (Figure 1) indicate that the main effect of G.A. is through shortening of the initial lag period. There was no change in cell size or generation time as a result of the G.A. in the medium.

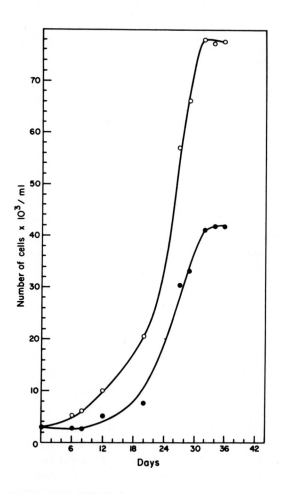

FIGURE 1.   Growth curves of *G. breve*
(o———o) with Gibberellic acid 10^{-7} M
(●———●) without Gibberellic acid

EXTRACTION OF TOXINS

Step 1

Cells from a 30 day culture (about 80,000 cells/ml) were collected by continuous flow centrifugation. The cells were lyophilized and the supernatant was discarded.

Step 2

Lyophilized cells were suspended in chloroform-methanol 2:1 (v/v). The slurry was homogenized, centrifuged, and the supernatant which contained the toxic principles was saved. This extraction procedure was repeated two more times and the cell pellet was extracted with pure methanol. All the supernatant fractions were combined, and the solvent was evaporated under vacuum.

Step 3

The dried residue was dissolved in a mixture of chloroform-methanol and water 8:2:1 (v/v). The mixture was shaken well and the two phases were then separated by a short centrifugation. The upper phase was removed and the lower organic phase which contained the toxic principle was washed again with the upper phase of the same solvent mixture.

Step 4

The lower organic phase was evaporated and the excess water was removed by dissolving the residue in Benzene-ethanol (4:1) followed by evaporation under vacuum.

Step 5

The material from Step 4 was mounted on a column of Sephadex LH-20 and fractionally eluted with chloroform-methanol 2:1 (v/v). Two active fractions were revealed, one neurotoxic and the other hemolytic (Figure 2). The fractions containing the bulk of each toxin were pooled, evaporated under vacuum and redissolved in methanol (10 mg/ml) for physiological experiments.

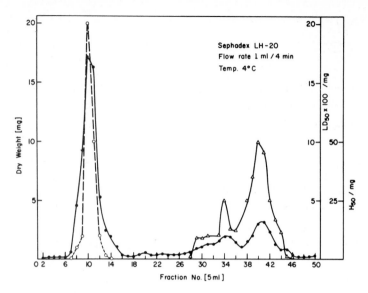

FIGURE 2.   Separation of neurotoxin (o ——— o) and hemolysin (△ ——— △) on sephadex LH-20. (● ——— ●) dry weight of fractionated toxin

BIOLOGICAL ACTIVITIES

The hemolytic activity was tested on washed rabbit red blood cells (Paster and Abbott, 1969). Lethal activity was determined by exposing *Gambusia affinis* minnows to serial dilutions of the toxin for 90 minutes. The specific activity was expressed as LD_{50} per milligram of solid.

We have recently reported (Paster and Abbott, 1969) that crude extracts of *G. breve* showed hemolytic activity in *vitro*. Using Sephadex LH-20 chromatography it is possible to separate the hemolytic fraction from the neurotoxic fraction.

The hemolytic fraction did not exhibit any lethal activity whereas the neurotoxic lethal fraction has several biological activities:

(1) Nerve conduction tested with the tibial nerve of *Rana pipiens* was blocked irreversibly at a low concentration (Figure 3).

(2) Intravenous injection of 150 μg toxin into the abdominal vein of *Rana pipiens* caused the heart to stop in diastole after a marked depolarization of the membrane and shortening of the action potential plateau of the heart muscle (Figure 4). There is usually a recovery from this effect after 5–6 minutes.

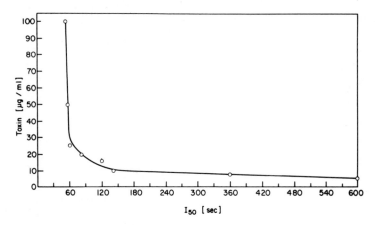

FIGURE 3.   Effect of the neurotoxic fractions on the tibial nerve of *Rana pipiens*. I_{50}, time in sec. needed to obtain 50% block of action potential

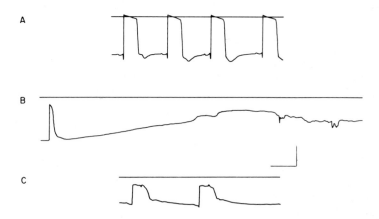

FIGURE 4.   Effect of the neurotoxic fractions on frog heart following injection of 150 µg toxin into abdominal vein. Calibrations 20 mv, 1 sec. A. control. B. 20 sec. after injection of toxin C. 6 min. after injection

(3) An increase in the beating rate of rat heart cells in tissue culture was observed when neurotoxin was added (Table 1).

(4) Injection of the neurotoxin in the intact vertebrates induces spontaneous contraction of the body musculature followed by a fatal paralysis. Martin and Chatterjee (1969) have reported that their preparations exhibit an anti-acetylcholinesterase activity and our findings of a shortened plateau of the

TABLE 1   Effect of neurotoxin from *G. breve* on heart cells* beating in tissue culture

Toxin (µg/ml)	Beating Rate** (no./min)
0.00	32 (3)
0.25	30 (3)
2.5	50 (5)
25	75 (5)
125	85 (3)

*8 days old,**2 min after application

heart electrogram and of spontaneous skeletal muscle contracture are not inconsistent with such anti-acetylcholinesterase activity (Burgen and Terroux, 1953)

The neurotoxic fraction can be separated into 4 active fractions using thin-layer chromatography. It appears from this separation that two of the active components are associated with a carotenoid moiety. We do not have enough information to determine whether this association occurs naturally in the cells, or is an associative artefact of extraction.

SUMMARY

Gymnodinium breve is a toxigenic marine dinoflagellate. Periodically this organism increases in number and discolors coastal waters, mainly along the eastern coast of the U.S.A. and the Gulf of Mexico, and the phenomenon popularly known as 'Red Tide' results.

We have found that Gibberellic acid (GA) stimulates the growth of *G. breve* in a synthetic medium containing inorganic salts, trace elements and three vitamins (thiamin-HCl 1 mg/L, biotin 0.5 µg/L, and B_{12} 1 µg/L). $10^{-7}M$ of GA gave the maximum effect while concentrations higher than $5 \times 10^{-7}M$ were inhibitory. In the absence of GA, there is a lag period of normally 6 to 8 days following innoculation. In the presence of GA this lag is abolished and the logarithmic phase of growth starts immediately. By adding the GA to the growth medium we were able to collect as much as $80 \cdot 10^6$ cells/L, in 30 days. These conditions have made available to us work quantities of cells adequate to elucidate the physiological action and to begin studies on the chemical structure of *G. breve* toxins.

By using a sequence of extraction procedures with chromatography on Sephadex LH-20, we were able to separate two different toxins: 1) a neurotoxin, which is lethal to fish, frogs and mice and 2) a hemolytic fraction which hemolyses red blood cells *in vitro*. The neurotoxin of *G. breve* blocks nerve conduction and increases the rate of heart beat in intact heart or cell culture up to blockage in diastole, in high dosage, without causing any visible cytological damage.

References

Burgen, A. S. V. and R. O. Terroux 1953 'On the negative isotropic effect of cat's auricle.' *J. Physiol.*, **120**: 449.

Cummins, J. M., A. A. Stevens, B. E. Huntley, F. W. Hill and J. W. Higgins 1967 'Some properties of *Gymnodinium breve* toxins determined bioanalytically in mice.' *In*: Freudenthal, H. D. (ed.), *Drugs from the Sea*. p. 213. The Marine Technology Society, Washington, D.C.

Martin, D. F. and A. B. Chatterjee 1969 'Isolation and characterization of a toxin from the Florida red tide organism.' *Nature*, **221**: 59.

McFarren, E. F., H. Tanabe, F. J. Silva, W. B. Wilson, J. E. Campbell and K. H. Lewis 1965 'The occurrence of a ciguatera-like poison in oysters, clams and *Gymnodinium breve* cultures.' *Toxicon*, **3**: 111.

Paster, Z. and B. C. Abbott 1969 'Hemolysis of rabbit erythrocytes by *Gymnodinium breve* toxin.' *Toxicon*, **7**: 245.

Ray, S. and D. V. Aldrich 1965 *Gymnodinium breve*: 'Induction of Shellfish poisoning in chicks.' *Science*, **148**: 1748.

Spikes, J. J., S. M. Ray, D. V. Aldrich and J. B. Nash 1968 'Toxicity variations of *Gymnodinium breve* cultures.' *Toxicon*, **5**: 171.

Wilson, W. B. and S. M. Ray 1956 'The occurrence of *Gymnodinium breve* in the Western Gulf of Mexico.' *Ecology*, **37**: 388.

WITHAFERIN A, A MITOTIC POISON ISOLATED FROM *WITHANIA SOMNIFERA* DUN

B. SHOHAT, S. GITTER and D. LAVIE

The Pharmacological Institute, The Rogoff-Wellcome Research Institute, Beilinson Hospital, Petah Tikva and the Department of Chemistry, The Weizmann Institute of Science, Rehovot, Israel

INTRODUCTION

DURING A SYSTEMATIC screening program of the Israeli flora for new antitumor compounds, withaferin A was isolated from the leaves of *Withania somnifera* Dun. (Solanaceae) (Lavie *et al.*, 1965, Shohat *et al.*, 1967). Kupchan *et al.* (1965) have also isolated the same compound from *Acnistus arborescens* L., a Solanaceae from Central America, and reported its tumor inhibitory action.

The present research deals with further investigations on the antitumor properties of withaferin A.

MATERIALS AND METHOD

Compound

Withaferin A, $C_{28}H_{38}O_6$ (Shohat *et al.*, 1967), was suspended in 0.85 NaCl solution containing 0.5 per cent carboxymethylcellulose. The approximate LD_{50} of the compound injected by the intraperitoneal route into Swiss mice weighing 18–22 g was established as 54 mg/kg mouse weight.

Experimental tumors

The experimental mouse tumors used in this study were S-180, sarcoma Black (SBL_1), EO771 mammary adenocarcinoma and Ehrlich ascites carcinoma (Lettré).

In vivo studies

Chemotherapy   Withaferin A was injected into tumor bearing animals 24 hrs after tumor implantation in the solid tumors. In the Ehrlich ascites tumor bearing mice, treatment was started 1, 24, 48, 72 hr or 5 and 7 days after tumor implantation. In the solid tumors injections were repeated every 24 hr during a period of 14 days. In the Ehrlich ascites tumor bearing mice one single or several daily doses of withaferin A were used. In all experiments withaferin A was given by the intraperitoneal route. The carcinostatic effect was determined according to specifications of the Cancer Chemotherapy National Service Center (1959).

Cytology and cytochemistry   Samples of ascites tumor cells were aspirated 2, 4, 24, 48 and 72 hr after withaferin A administration. From every sample, several smears were prepared and stained with Giemsa, by the Feulgen squash method for DNA, with methyl green pyronin for RNA and by Gomori's lead technique for acid phosphatase. The mitotic index which expresses the number of mitoses per 1000 cells counted was determined. Total tumor cells and total leukocyte counts of the ascitic fluid from the withaferin A treated mice were performed and compared to controls.

In vitro studies

Human malignant cells, pleural and peritoneal effusions from patients with advanced neoplastic diseases were used. The primary tumors of these patients were carcinomas of the ovary and carcinomas of the mammary gland. 3×10^6 cells in 3 ml medium were incubated for 24 hr at $37°$ C in a shaker with various concentrations of withaferin A. Following incubation a drop of the suspension was stained with 0.5 per cent eosin vital staining according to Schreck (1936).

PROCEDURES AND RESULTS

In vivo studies

Chemotherapy   Daily intraperitoneal injections of withaferin A at a dose of 10 mg/kg given for periods between 6–14 days, produced high significant growth retardation of the several tumors tested, and up to 100 per cent inhibition was observed for Ehrlich ascites carcinoma bearing mice (Shohat *et al.*, 1967) after receiving only one dose of withaferin A, if the compound was administered 24 or 48 hr after tumor transplantation. These 'cured' mice were found to be resistant to rechallenge (Shohat *et al.*, 1970).

Cytology and cytochemistry   A marked increase of the number of cells in metaphase in the treated Ehrlich ascites tumor bearing mice was observed as early as 4 hr after withaferin A administration (10 mg/kg). Microscopical examination of the arrested cells in the metaphase 4 hr after administration of the compound showed a picture of dividing cells with chromosomes irregularly scattered in the cell showing no equatorial arrangement. One could observe abnormal forms such as star, ball or exploded and agglutinated chromosomes (Plate I, Figures 1, 2, 3, 4).

Cytochemical tests for DNA and RNA showed no change in the distribution of these two constituents in the cell when compared to controls. Daily differential counts of the ascitic fluid obtained from the treated Ehrlich ascites bearing mice showed an increase in the polymorphonuclear population of the peritoneal cavity 24 hr after injection followed by an increase in the macrophage population and a decrease of tumor cells. The administration of a single dose of 25 or 40 mg of withaferin A/kg mouse weight, as well as daily repeated doses of 10 mg/kg, produced disappearance of the tumor cells within 3–6 days. The single doses mentioned were more effective than the repeated lower doses. In the same period control animals showed the usual development of the intraperitoneal tumor.

A marked accumulation of acid phosphatese granules especially in the macrophages surrounding the tumor cells was seen in the withaferin A treated samples. The tumor cells were found to be surrounded by the macrophages in rosette-like form only in the treated samples.

In vitro studies

The human malignant ascites cells or pleural tumor cells were incubated for 24 hr at 37° C in the nutrient medium TC 199 + 20 per cent human ascitic fluid with various concentrations of withaferin A. Incubation of these cells with 10 γ/ml for 24 hr at 37° C brought about 50 per cent of cell death. A higher concentration 20 γ/ml caused complete destruction of the tumor cells (Plate II, Figures 5, 6, 7, 8).

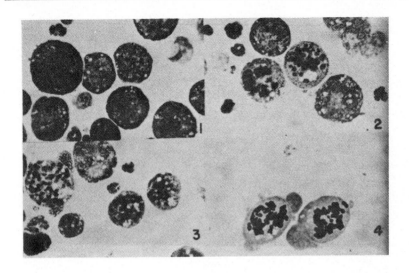

PLATE I   Photomicrographs of Ehrlich ascites tumor cells obtained from withaferin A treated mice. May-Grunwald Giemsa stained smears, X 1000

FIGURE 1.   Untreated control Ehrlich ascites carcinoma.

FIGURE 2.   Star and exploded metaphase 4 hr after i.p. administration of 10 mg/kg withaferin A

FIGURE 3.   Exploded metaphase as above

FIGURE 4.   Exploded and clumped chromosomes 4 hr after administration of 10 mg/kg withaferin A

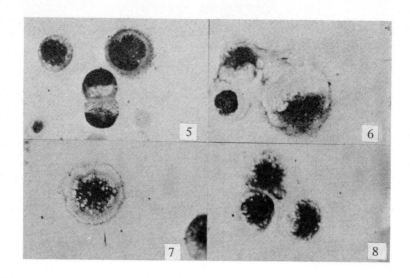

PLATE II   Human malignant cells from pleural effusions of a patient with mammary carcinoma stained by May-Grunwald Giemsa X 1000

FIGURE 5   Untreated human malignant cells after incubation of 24 hr at 37° C in medium.

FIGURES 6, 7, 8.   Withaferin A treated cells (10 γ/ml) after incubation as above. Dissolution of tumor cells is observed.

TOXICITY AND CARCINOGENIC ACTION IN RATS OF ELAIOMYCIN, A METABOLITE OF *STREPTOMYCES HEPATICUS*

R. SCHOENTAL

M.R.C. Toxicology Research Unit, M.R.C. Laboratories,
Carshalton, Surrey, England

INTRODUCTION

MOST OF THE POISONS discussed at this Toxinology Symposium, though they vary greatly in their chemical structures and mode of action, have in common the ability to cause acute poisoning with exceedingly small doses, almost 3 orders lower than those normally dealt with in Toxicology. There is, however, some overlapping as regards the size of the toxic dose (compare Table 1) and strict division between Toxinology and Toxicology is not possible.

Due to their often dramatic acute effects, venoms attracted attention already in antiquity and have been studied ever since. However, little attention has been paid to the investigation of chronic and possible carcinogenic effects, which some of these compounds may possess. There seems to be a general belief that recovery from an acute episode has no long lasting consequences. This belief was probably based on the observations that in man carcinogenic effects follow after prolonged, repeated exposure to carcinogenic agents, some of which are listed in Table 2. With most of these agents repeated treatment was usually required in order to induce tumours also in animals.

In the last 15 years, however, experiments in animals have shown that a *single* exposure to a carcinogenic agent may be sufficient to induce tumours which become apparent only after a long time interval. Examples of such

TABLE 1   Approximate toxicities of certain natural toxins

	μg/kg b.w.		mg/kg b.w.
Botulinus	0.00003	Amanitine	0.1
Tetanus	0.0001	Sporidesmin	0.25
Crotalus	0.2	Strychnine	0.5
Cobra	0.3	Phalloidine	2.0
Diphtheria	0.3	Noradrenalin*	5.0
Tetrodotoxin	10.0	Aflatoxin	10.0
Echinodermotoxin	20.0	Retrorsine	35.0
Physalistoxin	100.0	Elaiomycin	40.0
Serotonin*	300.0	Streptozotocin	100.0
Bufotoxin	400.0	Methionine*	750.0
Salamandrine	1000.0	Cycasin	1000.0

* Physiological constituents of tissues

TABLE 2   Examples of agents known to induce tumours in man and in experimental animals

Aromatic amines	Bladder cancer (Workers in the dye industry)
Polycyclic aromatic hydrocarbons	Scrotal cancer (Chimney sweeps)
Radioactive substances	Lung cancer (Joahimsthal miners)
	Oran cancer (Painters of luminous watch-dials)
Ultraviolet rays	Skin cancer (Australia)
X-rays	Leukaemia, etc. (Radiologists) (Children irradiated *in utero*)

carcinogens are among those listed in Table 3 and are marked by an asterisk. Of these, elaiomycin has been chosen to illustrate the hazard to man and animals from environmental natural products, and the variety of systemic lesions and tumours that can be induced even by a single dose of such a 'natural carcinogen (Schoental, 1969, 1970).

TABLE 3   Examples of agents which induce tumours in experimental animals
(* even with a single dose)

Natural	Synthetic
Aflatoxins*	Azo-dyes
Cycasin*	Alkylnitroso-compounds*
Elaiomycin*	Epoxides
Streptozotocin*	
Pyrrolizidine alkaloids*	
α, β-unsaturated lactones	
Viruses*	

Elaiomycin, the metabolite of *Streptomyces hepaticus* has been isolated
and studied in the laboratories of Park, Davis & Co., because *in vitro* it
appeared to have a tuberculostatic action. However, it proved rather toxic
and had no therapeutic effects against experimental infections in mice and
guinea-pigs. It caused liver cirrhosis in guinea-pigs on repeated dosage (20
mg/kg body weight/day s.c. 3–4 weeks) (Ehrlich *et al.*, 1954; Haskell *et al.*,
1954).

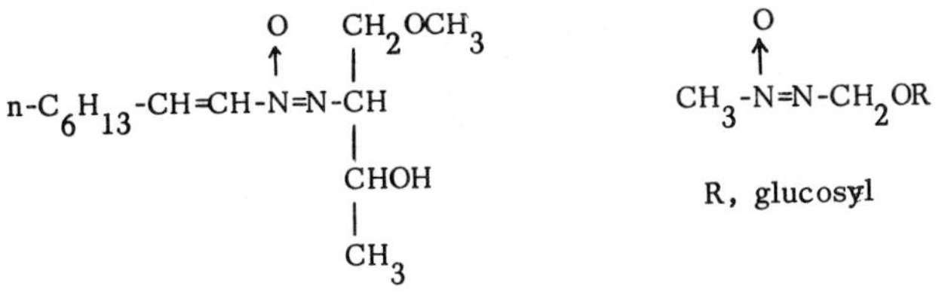

Elaiomycin

I

Cycasin

II

FIGURE 1.   Structures of elaiomycin and cycasin

The structure of elaiomycin has been elucidated by Stevens *et al.*, (1958).
It is 4-methoxy-3-(1-ctenyl-NON-azoxy)-2-butanol (Figure 1). In view of the
similarity to the carcinogenic cycasin (Laqueur and Spatz, 1968) (the gluco-
side of methylazoxymethanol (Figure 1 (II)) that has been isolated from nuts
of *Cycas circinalis* L, a palm-like tree growing on Guam), it was of interest to
test elaiomycin for carcinogenic activity.

MATERIALS AND METHODS

Through the courtesy of Dr. Ehrlich, a small quantity of elaiomycin was obtained from Parke, Davis & Co. This proved to cause liver necrosis not only in mice, but also in rats. The latter were mostly used for the study of chronic effects.

White rats, derived from the Porton Strain, bred randomly in the M.R.C. Laboratories, Carshalton, were used for chronic studies. Elaiomycin as an emulsion in aqueous ethanol or in arachis oil was administered by stomach tube to weanlings, and by s.c. or i.p. injection to male and female rats one or a few days old (referred to as 'newly-borns'). The latter were returned to their mothers, having been kept separately for 30 minutes in order to prevent her licking off the material from the site of injection. At weaning, the rats were separated according to sex and kept in metal cages, about 5 rats per cage. The rats were weighed at the beginning of the experiment and at monthly intervals or more often. Both mothers and weanling rats were given the normal diet MRC 41B and water *ad libitum*. All the animals that died or that were killed by coal gas when they appeared ill, were autopsied, the livers, lungs, stomach, kidneys and any other organs which seemed abnormal were fixed in Helly or neutral 10% formol saline solution; sections cut at 5–6 μ were stained routinely with haematoxylin and eosin for microscopic examination. Other stains were used when required.

RESULTS AND DISCUSSION

The experiments were performed on 28 male and 24 female weanling white rats and on 30 male and 29 female newly-born ones. Doses of elaiomycin in excess of 40 mg/kg killed the animals within a few days. Microscopically, the main lesions included centrilobular liver necrosis, lung congestion, tubular damage in the kidneys, and congestion and ulceration of the stomach.

Among rats which received smaller doses, most survived for more than 1½ years and some developed tumours. The incidence of tumours was higher in rats which had several doses, though the dosage was obviously not optimal for a high incidence of tumours. Table 4 summarises the survival times and the dosage of the rats which had significant lesions and multiple tumours. Such tumours have not been seen in our control rats.

As elaiomycin, a metabolite of a soil organism (*Streptomyces hepaticus*),

TABLE 4   Survival times and dosage of rats that developed multiple chronic lesions and tumours after elaiomycin

Sex	Age at 1st dose	Survival time after 1st dose (months)	No. & size of doses (mg/kg b.w.)	Route	Lesions and Tumours
♀	n	18K	20	s.c.	Adenocarcinoma of stomach; pituitary tumour
♂	n	19½K	25 + 10	s.c.	Tumour of thymus and of salivary gland
♀	n	21K	20	s.c. or i.p.	Squamous carcinoma of Fallopian tube; glandular stomach hyperplasia
♀	n	23½K	20	s.c. or i.p.	Stomach adenoma; uterine adenoma; pituitary tumour
♂	n	28K	25 + 20 + 10 + 10	s.c.	Adenoma of pancreas; pituitary tumour
♂	n	29k	25 + 20 + 10 + 10	s.c.	Rhabdomyosarcoma; adenoma of stomach
♂	n	29K	25 + 20 + 10 + 10	s.c. or i.p.	Liver sarcoma; pancreatic adenoma
♂	n	30K	20 + 20		Mesothelioma of testes; pituitary tumour
♂	w	27D	26 + 4 + 25 + 25	oral + i.p.	Adenocarcinoma of kidney
♂	w	28K	26 + 10 + 5	oral	Widely spread reticulum cell tumour; thymic tumour
♂	w	28K	35	oral	Sarcoma; stomach ulcer
♂	w	28K	35,	oral	Brain tumour; stomach ulcer; bladder concretions
♂	w	28K	35	oral	Liver sarcoma; stomach hyperplasia; brain tumour.

D—died
K—killed
n—'newly-born,' one or a few days old
w—weanling

proved to be carcinogenic for several tissues of the rat, in which it induced the types of tumours which are seen in man, its detection in human environment becomes necessary. In many parts of the world, grain foods are stored in underground pits, in direct contact with the soil, where contamination

TABLE 5   Annual mortality rates per 100,000 persons aged 45–64 years, standardized for age (for 1960–1) (R. Doll, J. Natl. Cancer Inst., 1967)

	Cancer of the							
	Oesophagus		Stomach		Colon		Rectum	
	M	F	M	F	M	F	M	F
England & Wales	6.9	4.0	49.9	20.2	19.4	21.6	14.8	9.8
Japan	13.3	4.1	153.1	78.3	5.2	5.4	7.7	7.1
U.S.A. (white)	7.3	1.6	18.7	8.7	22.3	24.8	10.6	7.4
U.S.A. (non-white)	24.7	6.5	44.4	19.6	21.2	26.4	10.7	9.5
Russian S.F.S.R.	16.0	6.5	128.5	-66.2			5.8	5.7
Turkmenian S.S.R.	72.8	75.5	110.0	46.7				
Variation factor	10.5	47.0	8.0	9.7	4.5	4.9	2.6	1.7

with *Streptomyces* metabolites is conceivable. It has to be noted that elaiomycin has been isolated not only from the strain of *Streptomyces* found in Ohio, U.S.A., but also from organisms found in soil in Japan (Ohkuma *et al.*, 1957). In Japan the incidence of stomach cancer is very high (Table 5) and is often associated with stomach ulcers (Oota, 1968). Glandular stomach tumours have been reported in a small proportion of rats given diets containing aflatoxins (the metabolites of *Aspergillus flavus*), but these were not connected with stomach ulcers (Butler and Barnes, 1966).

For the detection of elaiomycin in foodstuffs, the methods used for the isolation of aflatoxin from groundnut meals can be adopted in conjunction with gas-liquid chromatography (GLC). GLC proved a convenient method not only for the detection and estimation of elaiomycin, but also of its decomposition products. (Mr. S. Gibbard, personal communication).

Streptomyces and actinomyces are microorganisms widely distributed in Nature. They have been extensively studied, but mainly as sources of antibiotics; among their metabolites have been found many valuable drugs, which are now in use for chemotherapy (Miller, 1961). The structures of the various metabolites so far known, vary considerably—many are macrolides and polypeptides, but some, like elaiomycin and streptozotocin are relatively simple chemical compounds.

Streptozotocin, the metabolite of *Streptomyces achromogens* has been isolated and studied in the laboratories of the Upjohn Company. Its structure (Herr *et al.*, 1967) is related to the carcinogenic alkylnitrosamides, (Figure 2) while elaiomycin is an α, β-unsaturated alkylazoxy compound, related to cycasin (Figure 1).

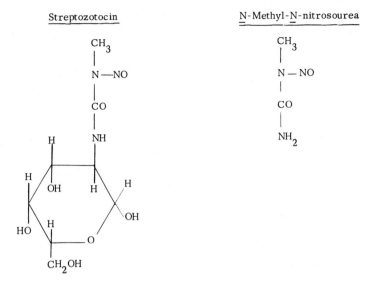

FIGURE 2.   Structures of streptozotocin and *N*-methyl-*N*-nitrosourea

Streptozotocin has been used for chemotherapy of tumours before its diabetogenic (Rakieten *et al.*, 1963) and carcinogenic action has been recognised. With a single dose it can induce tumours in rat kidney (Arison and Feudale, 1967); liver tumours including liver sarcoma have been induced in hamsters (Sibay and Hayes, 1969). Carcinogenic effects have also been reported for actinomycins K. L. and S. (Kawamata *et al.* 1959) (quoted by Kraybill and Shimkin, 1964). These examples illustrate the need for testing for chronic effects of metabolites of streptomyces and actinomyces as well as many other 'natural' products that show acute toxicity.

The possible relevance of 'natural' toxins for the aetiology of chronic diseases and tumours in animal and man has been recognised, and no doubt more such examples will soon be found in human environment.

SUMMARY

Elaiomycin (4-methoxy-3-(1-octenyl-NON-azoxy)-2-butanol) a metabolite of *Streptomyces hepaticus*, caused liver necrosis and death in young rats given doses in excess of 40 mg/kg body weight. Smaller doses allowed the animals to survive for long periods up to 2½ years. A variety of lesions and tumours were found among the surviving rats: testicular atrophy, gastric ulcers, adenoma and adenocarcinoma of the pyloric region of the stomach, adenoma of the kidney, of the small intestine, of the exocrine pancreas, liver sarcoma, brain oligodendroglioma and thymic and lymphoid tumours. Even single doses were effective, though tumours were more numerous when multiple doses were given. The types of tumours resemble those seen in man, some of which can be induced also by cycasin or by streptozotocin. The possibility has to be considered that such 'natural products' may play a part in the aetiology of human cancer.

References

Arison, R. N. and E. L. Feudale 1967 'Induction of renal tumour by streptozotocin in rats.' *Nature*, **214**: 1254–1255.

Butler, W. H. and J. M. Barnes 1966 'Carcinoma of the glandular stomach in rats given diets containing aflatoxins.' *Nature*, 209: 90.

Ehrlich, J., L. E. Anderson, G. L. Coffey, W. H. Feldman, M. W. Fisher, A. B. Hillegas, A. G. Karlson, M. P. Kundsen, J. K. Weston, A. S. Youmans and G. P. Youmans 1954 'Elaiomycin, a new tuberculostatic antibiotic.' *Antibiot. Chemotherapy*, 4: 338–342.

Haskell, T. H., A. Ryder and Q. R. Bartz 1954 'Elaiomycin, a new tuberculostatic antibiotic.' *Antibiot. Chemotherapy*, 4: 141–144.

Herr, R. R., H. K. Jahnke and A. D. Argoudelis 1967 'The structure of streptozotocin.' *J. Am. Chem. Soc.*, 89: 4808–4809.

Kawamata, J., N. Nakabayashi, A. Kawai, H. Fujita, M. Imanishi and R. Ikegami 1959 'Carcinogenic effects of actinomycin.' *Biken J.*, 2: 105–112.

Kraybill, H. F. and M. B. Shimkin 1964 'Carcinogenesis related to foods contaminated by processing and fungal metabolites.' *Advan. Cancer Res.*, 8: 191–248.

Laqueur, G. L. and M. Spatz 1968 'Toxicology of Cycasin.' *Cancer Res.*, **28**: 2262–2267.

Miller, M. W. 1961 *The Pfizer Handbook of Microbial Metabolites*. McGraw Hill, New York.

Ohkuma, K., G. Nakamura and S. Yamashita 1957 'An antibiotic produced by Streptomyces strain No. 1252, identical with elaiomycin.' *J. Antibiotics (Japan), Ser. A.*, 10: 224–225.

Oota, K. 1968 'On the nature of the ulcerative changes in early carcinoma of the stomach.' *Gann Monograph*, 3: 141–151.

Rakieten, N., M. L. Rakieten and M. V. Nadkarni 1963 'The diabetogenic action of streptozotocin (NSC-37917).' *Cancer Chemotherapy Rep.*, 29: 91–98.

Schoental, R. 1969 'Carcinogenic action of elaiomycin.' *Nature*, 221: 765–766.

Schoental, R. 1970 'Gastric lesions including adenocarcinoma of the glandular stomach induced in rats by elaiomycin, a metabolite of *Streptomyces hepaticus.*' *Gann Monograph*, 8. (In press).

Sibay, T. M. and J. A. Hayes 1969 'Potential carcinogenic effect of streptozotocin.' *Lancet*, 2: 912.

Stevens, C. L., B. T. Gillis, J. C. French and T. H. Haskell 1958 'Elaiomycin. An aliphatic α, β-unsaturated azoxy compound.' *J. Am. Chem. Soc.*, 80: 6088–6092.

ETUDE THEORIQUE ET EXPERIMENTALE DE LA FIXATION DES TOXIQUES ET DES MEDICAMENTS SUR LES MACROMOLECULES PROTEIQUES

O. G. CESAIRE, F. FAURAN, M. J. FAURAN-CLAVEL

Laboratoires de Chimie analytique et Toxicologie de la
Faculté mixte de Médecine et Pharmacie de l'Université
de Dakar, Senegal

L'ADSORPTION et la désorption d'un médicament ou d'un toxique susceptible de se fixer sur les protéines du plasma sanguin, peuvent être décisives dans la mesure où ces phénomènes déterminent l'intégration plus ou moins réversible d'une substance étrangère dans le milieu intérieur. C'est en effet de la fraction non fixée de la substance étrangère que peut dépendre son action immédiate, l'action différée étant en revanche sous la dépendance de l'évolution du complexe protéine-substance éxogène. Le cas le plus typique de cette modulation de l'activité médicamenteuse est celui des barbituriques où il est possible, en outre, d'établir une relation entre la fixation sur les protéines plasmatiques et des caractères purement structuraux. La formation difficilement réversible d'un complexe protéine-toxique peut aussi expliciter les propriétés cumulatives de certains poisons, notamment ceux du groupe des 'thioloprives.'

Ces considérations tendent à faire jouer au support protéique le rôle statique d'un régulateur de l'activité médicamenteuse ou toxique. On peut concevoir également un rôle dynamique de la protéine pouvant se manifester par ses comportements immunologiques ou biochimiques.

La substance chimique étant un haptène, le complexe protéine-toxique, peut induire la formation d'un anticorps susceptible de révéler ses potentialités lors d'une administration ultérieure de toxique.

Parmi les conséquences biochimiques de la fixation du toxique ou du médicament sur les protéines, nous signalerons trois phénomènes: inhibition ou modulation de l'activité biocatalytique si le support protéique constitue un enzyme; déplacement de certains composés biologiquement actifs (histamine, sérotonine, bilirubine) par le simple jeu d'une compétition du médicament ou du poison pour l'occupation du site habituel de fixation; création de sites protéiques nouveaux particulièrement réactifs, à la suite de la génese sur la protéine d'une fonction chimique nouvelle due à l'interaction protéine-toxique.

Ces importantes notions sont d'une grande actualité et R. Truhaut (1965), a passé en revue il y a quatre ans les modalités et les conséquences de la fixation sur les protéines des principaux toxiques minéraux et organiques.

Les principales études théoriques tendant à définir les lois qui régissent l'interaction des substances chimiques sur les protéines apparaissent en 1948 avec les travaux de G. Scatchard (1949), Scatchard et Black (1949) puis de T. R. Hugues et I. M. Klotz (1960). Compte tenu du fait que la première étape d'une réaction enzymatique est la formation intermédiaire d'un complexe protéine-substrat (protéine-inhibiteur ou protéine-activateur) par le jeu d'une combinaison théorique, J. Monod et al., (1963) élaborent quelques années plus tard la théorie de la régulation allostérique des systèmes enzymatiques. Koshland et ses collaborateurs (1966) devaient récemment proposer un 'modèle' susceptible de justifier les anomalies expérimentales observées dans l'étude cinétique de certains systèmes enzymatiques (cinétiques dites non Michaeliennes).

L'adsorption sur les protéines catalytiquement actives d'une substance biogène—co-enzyme, produit intermédiaire ou terminal d'une chaîne métabolique ou d'un composé exogène—médicament ou toxique—peut donc être mise en évidence par une modulation de l'activité enzymatique en présence de substrat. Elle se traduira par une cinétique particulière de la transformation de celui-ci. Nous pensons qu'il s'agit là d'un cas particulier de l'étude expérimentale de la fixation sur des macromolécules envisagées, du point de vue de ses conséquences enzymologiques car les protéines structurales ne sont pas justiciables d'une telle méthode d'étude. Nous n'examinerons par conséquent dans l'exposé qui va suivre que des techniques générales s'appliquant aux protéines structurales comme aux protéines enzymatiques et permettant de définir les conditions stoechiométriques de la formation des complexes protéine-substance chimique.

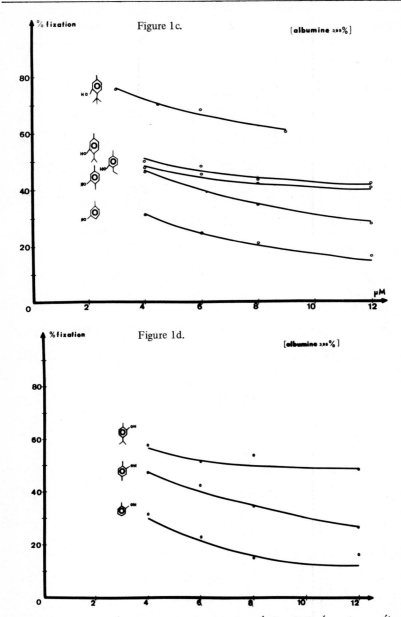

FIGURE 1.   Etude expérimentale de la fixation des crésols substitués sur les protéines sériques d'après

FAURAN *et al.* (1967)

La fixation de ces dérivés a été étudiés sur du sérum bovin total (1a et 1b), puis sur la seuls fraction albuminique en quantité équivalente à celle contenue dans les essais précédents (1c *m* 1d)

mentales de F et de C. Pour chaque couple on déduira facilement une valeur de r égale au rapport du nombre de molécules toxique lié au nombre de molécules de protéine.

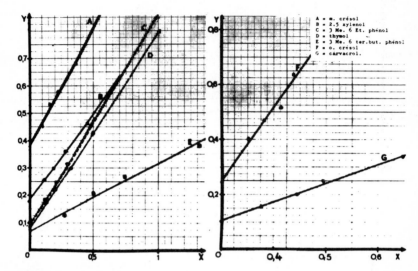

FIGURE 2.   Application de la transformation graphique de KLOTZ au cas de certains crésols

substitués d'aprés FAURAN (1968).

Les résultats expérimentaux obtenus précédemment (voir graphiques 1c et 1d) ont été étudiés en utilisant la transformation graphique de KLOTZ (voir texte):

– en ordonnée on a porté $\frac{1}{r}$ (nombre de molécules de protéine/nombre de moles de toxique lié),

– en abscisse $\frac{1}{T}$ (inverse du nombre de molécules de toxique libre)

$$r = \frac{\frac{CF}{100}}{M_T} \cdot \frac{M_p}{P} = \frac{CF\,M_p}{100\,P\,M_T} \qquad \text{(VIII)}$$

ainsi qu'un nombre de molécules de toxique libre T:

$$T = \frac{(100-F)\,C}{100\,M_T} \qquad \text{(IX)}$$

Dès lors une étude graphique permettra de calculer n et K. Parmi les nombreuses méthodes proposées nous retiendrons celles indiquées respectivement par Klotz et Scatchard (cf. Hugues et Klotz, 1960).

Transformation graphique de Klotz   Dans la méthode de Klotz on étudiera graphiquement les variations de $\dfrac{1}{r}$ en fonction de l'inverse du nombre de molécules de toxique libre $=\dfrac{1}{T}$.

Si nous sommes dans le cas théorique défini par l'équation III: (sites indépendants et équivalents) la relation

$$r = \frac{n\,KT}{1 + KT} \text{ peut aussi s'écrire } \frac{1}{r} = \frac{1}{nKT} + \frac{1}{n} \tag{X}$$

La courbe représentative des variations de $\dfrac{1}{r}$ en fonction de $\dfrac{1}{T}$ sera donc une droite (voir graphique no. 2) dont:

–l'ordonnée à l'origine est égale à $\dfrac{1}{n}$ d'où la détermination expérimentale de (n)

–la pente est égale à $\dfrac{1}{nK}$, d'où, connaissant n, le calcul possible de la valeur de K.

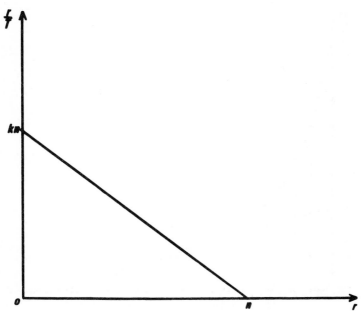

FIGURE 3.   Transformation graphique de Scatchard

Transformation graphique de Scatchard Scatchard a étudié les variations de $\frac{r}{T}$ en fonction de r. Si nous sommes dans le cas défini par l'equation III on peut écrire:

$$r + rKT = n\, k\, T$$
$$rKT - nKT = r \tag{XI}$$
$$\text{d'où}\, \frac{r}{T} = -nK + rK$$

par conséquent la courbe représentative de la fonction (XI) est une droite qui coupe l'axe des ordonnées à une ordonnée égale à Kn et l'axe des abcisses à une abcisse égale à n (voir graphique no. 3).

Interêt pratique des transformations graphiques La forme des courbes obtenues par l'une ou l'autre des deux transformations graphiques permet de déterminer les modalités de la fixation du toxique sur les sites récepteurs (sites équivalents et indépendants, sites équivalents mais non indépendants, plusieurs types de sites équivalents). Par exemple dans le cas d'une fixation mettant en jeu 2 types de sites équivalents, la transformation de Scatchard ne conduira plus à une droite (voir graphique no. 4). Compte tenu de l'équation

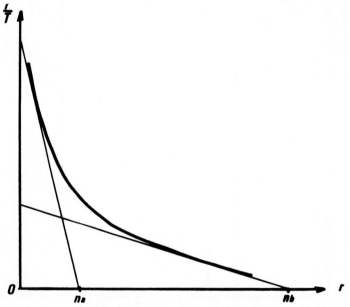

FIGURE 4.   Représentation graphique des résultats de la fixation d'une substance chimique sur une protéine dans le cas d'une interaction mettant en jeu deux types de sites équivalents (méthode graphique de Scatchard)

(VI), on déterminera à l'aide des 2 tangentes les couples de paramètres n_a K_a et n_b K_b définissant les modalités de l'interaction.

L'expression et la comparaison des résultats deviennent aussi possibles à l'intérieur d'une série chimique ou d'un auteur à un autre. Un résultat exprimé en pourcentage de fixation implique la précision de la nature de la protéine, sa quantité (P), la quantité de toxique mise en oeuvre (C), la force ionique du milieu, la température.

Outre la signification physique propre de ces valeurs, l'expression des résultats par 'n' et 'K' ne nécessite que la précision du type de protéine étudié, la force ionique du milieu et la température. La comparaison des résultats devient alors possible, ce qui accroît l'intérêt pratique de ces transformations graphiques.

2. TECHNIQUES D'ETUDE DE LA FIXATION DES TOXIQUES SUR LES MACROMOLECULES PROTEIQUES

Cette étude peut porter sur le milieu réactionnel global comportant, outre la protéine ayant fixé une fraction du toxique, la fraction libre de ce dernier. C'est essentiellement sur la détermination des variations de paramètres physiques spécifiques de la pròtéine princeps que portera l'analyse: spectres U.V. ou de fluorescence, paramètre électrochimique.

Dans d'autres cas l'analyse porte exclusivement sur la fraction libre du toxique et les problèmes analytiques se résument à l'étude des techniques permettant la séparation des molécules protéiques des petites molécules du toxique. Si pendant fort longtemps, parmi ces techniques, la dialyse a constitué la méthode de référence, il n'est est plus de même aujord'hui, la filtration sur gel, grâce en particulier à la modification apportée par Hummel et Dreyer, (1962) est plus volontiers employée à cause de sa rapidité et de sa spécificité.

Technique reposant sur l'etude globale du milieu reactionnel

La formation du complexe (P.T.) va retentir le plus souvent sur certains paramètres physicochimiques qui, s'ils étaient spécifiques de la protéine princeps (P), ne le seront plus pour le complexe (PT).

On peut determiner ces changements en utilisant soit des méthodes spectrales soit des en mesurant certains paramètres éléctrochimiques.

Changements spectraux

Spectres ultraviolets   La formation des complexes peut conduire à une modification de la position d'un maximum d'absorption ou de la valeur du coefficient d'extinction spécifique des protéines initiales. Pour la plupart d'entre elles, en effet, on peut disposer de spectres de référence (Beaven et Holiday, 1952). C'est ainsi que l'interaction du cuivre sur l'albumine bovine se traduit par une réduction de l'intensité de la bande de 375 nm, phénomène attribué à l'interaction des groupements sulfhydriles sur le cation bivalent (Hugues et Klotz, 1960). Ce même métal se fixe sur le DNA dénaturé, par un mécanisme différent mais l'observation du phenomène peut être faite d'une façon

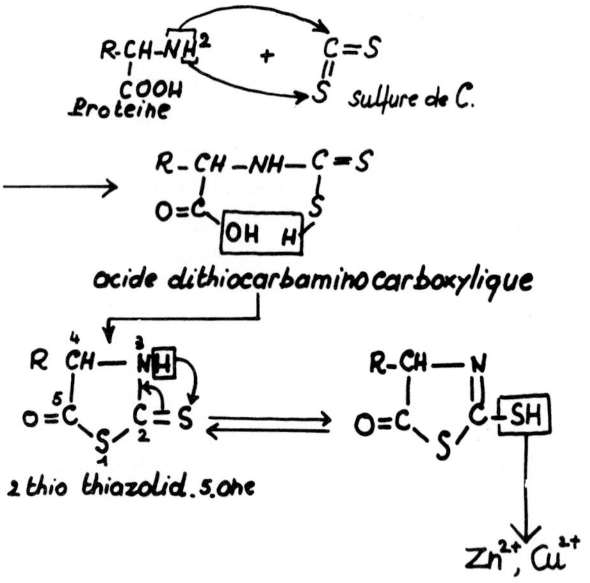

FIGURE 5.   Mécanisme de l'interaction du sulfure de carbone avec les protéines

analogue en U.V. (Eichhorn *et al.*, 1966). Dans le cas du sulfure de carbone (Truhaut, 1966), les modifications des positions du maximum d'absorption rendent compte des différentes étapes de la réaction (voir graphique no. 5).

Dans un premier temps la formation d'un acide dithiocarbaminocarboxylique se traduit par l'apparition d'un maximum à 250 et 290 nm. Sa cyclisation en 2 thio-thiazolid-5-one se traduit par un maximum à 280 nm. La forme tautomère de la 2-thio-thiazolid-5-one en se combinant aux ions Zn^{2+} et Cu^{2+} rend compte des manifestations histopathologiques de cette intoxication consécutives à la décroissance de la concentràtion cérébrale et sanguine par ces deux métaux.

Spectres de fluorescence   L'interaction d'une petite molécule avec une macromolécule protéique se traduit généralement par une décroissance de l'intensité de la fluorescence de la protéine pour un même système de longueur d'onde d'émission et d'excitation ('Quenching de fluorescence') (Salvatore *et al.*, 1966). Plus exceptionnellement, on a pu mettre en évidence une exaltation de la fluorescence de la protéine. A cet égard, il convient de citer les travaux de Löber (1964) sur les interactions du DNA sur l'orange d'acridine.

Dans tous ces éxemples, la stoechiométrie de la réaction pour une concentration donnée en protéine, peut être calculée en étudiant la variation du paramètre spectral en fonction de la concentration molaire en substance chimique. On obtient une courbe représentative des résultats d'allure hyperbolique à partir de laquelle par construction graphique, on détermine le point d'équivalence (C_S) (voir graphique no. 6).

Variation des parametres electrochimiques   La fixation de toxique ionisé sur les protéines peut dans certains cas conduire à des complexes dont la charge va être différente de celle de la protéine princeps. Cette variation pourra être mise en évidence par des mesures portant sur:
—la mobilité des protéines dans un champ électrique (électrophorèse),
—la conductivité globale de la solution,
—la f.e.m. de la solution (potentiométrie)
—le pH au cours de la titration de la protéine (Eichhorn *et al.*, 1966; Salvatore *et al.*, 1966).

Le plus souvent ces techniques ne permettent d'obtenir que des informations qualitatives, la présence simultanée de l'ion toxique libre et des complexes rendant difficile la détermination de la contribution de chacun d'eux au phénomène global.

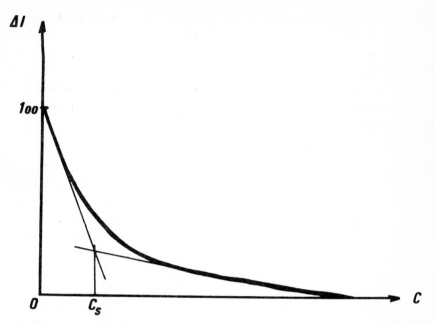

FIGURE 6.   Etude de la variation relative d'intensite de fluorescence d'une protéine en fonction de la concentration en substance chimique. Détermination de la stoechiométrie de la réaction

L'étude polarographique du courant de diffusion dans le milieu réactionnel pourrait conduire à une étude quantitative. En effet la diminution de ce courant apprécié en fonction de quantité de protéine ajoutée au milieu ne rend compte que de la quantité de toxique électroréductible, c'est-à-dire libre. Cependant les résultats sont toujours entachés d'erreur inhérentes à:

—l'adsorption de la protéine sur l'electrode
—la modification de la viscosité du milieu.

Techniques reposant sur l'analyse de la fraction libre du toxique apres separation des elements proteiques

La stoechiométrie de la formation du complexe ne peut être déterminée d'habitude par l'étude globale du milieu réactionnel et il est nécessaire le plus souvent d'effectuer la séparation préalable de la fraction libre du toxique du milieu protéique. Son évaluation ultérieure permettra de déterminer facilement le pourcentage de fixation, compte tenu soit de la quantité de toxique mise en oeuvre, soit de la quantité de toxique restant dans le milieu protéique.

Plusieurs procédés de séparation sont utilisables: l'électrophorèse, la centrifugation, la dialyse (statique ou dynamique), l'ultracentrifugation, l'ultrafiltration et la filtration sur gel.

Electrophorèse   C'est la technique la moins précise (Meunier, 1961). On réalise simultanément trois essais sur papier: (A) la protéine seule, (B) le toxique seul et (C) la protéine en présence du toxique.

L'essai (A) est révélé par l'amidoschwarz. Les essais (B) et (C) sont découpés en bandelettes de longueur égale et sont élués dans un solvant du toxique. Dans ces éluats, le toxique sera ensuite dosé (graphique no. 7). Ainsi l'on pourra déterminer, lorsqu'il s'agit d'un mélange complexe (plasma, sérum), la nature de la fraction protéine réceptrice, la quantité libre et la quantité fixée de toxique.

Il faudra éventuellement déceler aussi une mobilité différente du complexe par rapport à la protéine initiale en révélant un autre essai du type C par l'amidoschwarz.

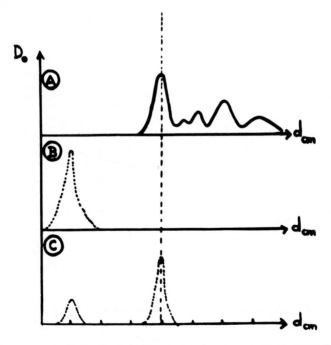

FIGURE 7.   Etude de la fixation d'un toxique sur les proteines plasmatiques par électrophorése

Cette technique rencontre deux grosses difficultés: le dépôt étant de l'ordre de 10 μl, la précision est faible; le dosage du toxique après élution exige l'emploi de techniques analytiques très sensibles.

Ultracentrifugation   C'est une technique précieuse pour l'étude de la fixation d'un composé chimique sur une protéine. On prépare à l'intérieur du tube à centrifuger du rotor un gradient de concentration en toxique et en protéine (l'utilisation d'un appareil à former les gradients est particulièrement indiquée). La centrifugation est réalisée à 200,000 g pendant plusieurs heures. Le tube à centrifuger est alors percé à sa base au moyen d'un 'perforateur de tube,' et le milieu recueilli à l'aide d'un collecteur de fraction. L'analyse porte à la fois sur la détermination de la concentration en protéine et sur celle èn toxique de chaque fraction. Si graphiquement on étudie la variation de ces deux paramètres, l'intersection par l'extrapolation de la droite avec l'axe des concentrations en toxique donne la quantité de toxique libre (graphique no. 8).

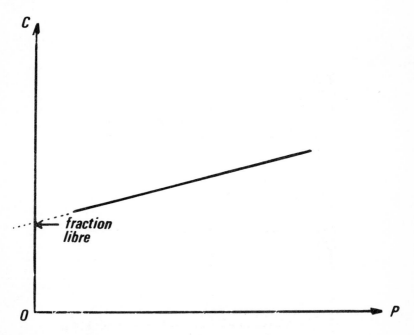

FIGURE 8.   Détermination de la fraction non fixée (T) par ultracentrifugation
En ordonnée : C = concentration en toxique ou médicament
P = concentration en protéine

A côté de ce premier pôle d'intérêt, l'ultracentrifugation, en permettant la détermination du poids moléculaire des protéines, peut parfois conduire à la mise en évidence d'associations protéiques intermoléculaires, telles que celles par exemple résultant de l'action des ions mercuriques sur les groupements thiols de la sérum albumine (P-S-Hg-S-P).

Parmi les études réalisées par ultracentrifugation, les travaux de Kersten *et al.* (1966) font ressortir la possibilité d'utiliser aussi bien les variations de la densité de flottation que celles du coefficient de sédimentation en fonction de la quantité utilisée de substances toxiques ou médicamenteuses. Cependant les résultats de ces auteurs n'ont été exploités qu'à des fins qualitatives.

Dialyse statique et dynamique   La dialyse utilise les propriétés de certaines membranes synthétiques (boyaux de cellulose Wisking) qui sont imperméables aux macromolécules comme les protéines mais perméables aux molécules de taille inférieure au diamètre de leurs pores (24 Å pour les membranes LKB).

Dans la dialyse statique, la protéine en solution tamponnée et la substance à étudier sont introduites dans le sac de dialyse (voir graphique no. 9) (Duggan et Luck, 1948; Scatchard et Black, 1949; Hugues et Klotz, 1960; Meunier,

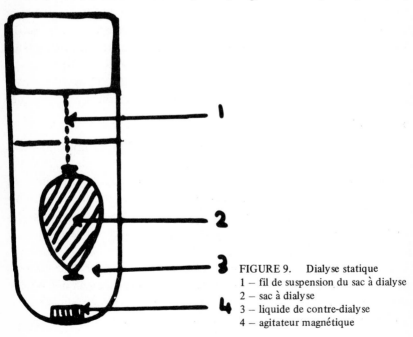

FIGURE 9.   Dialyse statique
1 — fil de suspension du sac à dialyse
2 — sac à dialyse
3 — liquide de contre-dialyse
4 — agitateur magnétique

1961; Stafford, 1962a; Fauran *et al.*, 1967a). L'opération s'effectue généralement à + 4° C afin d'éviter toute dénaturation de la protéine, cependant qu'une agitation manuelle ou mécanique augmente la vitesse de diffusion des particules dialysables. Initialement nulle, la concentration dans le compartiment externe de la substance à étudier va croître et tendre vers un état d'équilibre qui sera réalisé lorsque le nombre de molécules dialysables sera égal des deux côtés de la membrane. Toute variation du nombre de ces molécules dans le compartiment central consécutive en particulier à une fixation par la matériel protéique, se reflètera sur l'équilibre final et la composition du milieu externe. Il sera donc possible de rendre quantitativement compte de la fixation de la substance par un dosage de celle-ci dans chaque compartiment. Une telle technique nécessite donc un moyen de titration dans un milieu protéique (compartiment interne) ce qui parfois peut être délicat; aussi beaucoup d'auteurs préfèrent-ils utiliser la méthode dite de 'comparaison directe' (Meunier, 1961).

Pour chaque 'tube protéique' c'est-à-dire contenant une solution médicamenteuse et protéique, on réalise un tube dit 'non protéique' où l'on a mis au lieu à la place de la solution protéique une quantité équivalente de sérum physiologique ou de tampon avec la substance chimique étudiée.

Lorsque l'équilibre est atteint, le dosage du toxique dans le compartiment externe (dialysat) des deux essais permet de rendre compte du taux de fixation. Si la méthode de dosage repose sur une détermination spectrophotométrique, la densité optique suivra une variation linéaire en fonction de la concentration de la substance étudiée. Si Do est la densité optique correspondant au dosage de l'essai non protéique, Dp la densité optique mesurée pour l'essai protéique, on aura: Fixation % = $\dfrac{Do - Dp}{Do}$. 10^2 .

Deux sources d'erreurs entachent des mesures faites par utilisation de la dialyse:

—l'effet Donan peut entraîner une certaine asymétrie dans la distribution de corps qui sont des électrolytes forts; dans un tel cas, il faut apporter des corrections aux résultats numériques. Cependant, pour des électrolytes faibles (et c'est le cas des phénols), le phénomène est reconnu négligeable par Hugues et Klotz (1960).

—l'adsorption de la substance par la trame macromoléculaire de la cellulose du sac à dialyse peut être considérée comme une source d'erreur non négligeable. Mais on peut concevoir que dans la méthode de comparaison directe le phénomène n'a qu'une importance minime dans la mesure où il a lieu d'une façon identique dans le 'tube protéique' et dans le 'tube non protéique.'

Dans la dialyse dynamique, le compartiment externe du système est remplacé par un flux continu et à débit constant du liquide de contre-dialyse (voir graphique no. 10). De ce fait la loi exponentielle de diffusion des particules du toxique libre est modifiée. Globalement on observe donc une diminution du temps d'équilibre; néanmoins sa réalisation pratique ne se prête guère à la réalisation de séries (Seegers, 1943; Remenant, 1966; Vo Phi Hung, 1966; Chambon *et al.*, 1968).

Ultrafiltration   De même que la dialyse, l'ultrafiltration utilise les propriétés de semi-perméabilité de certaines membranes. Cependant, contrairement à la dialyse, la séparation des milieux protéiques de la phase aqueuse contenant le toxique libre est complète et réalisée par l'intermédiaire d'une dépression permettant la seule filtration des petites molécules (Thorp, 1964). Les principaux inconvénients sont: les modifications quantitatives du complexe soumis à une dépression importante; l'adsorption des protéines par la trame de l'ultrafiltre; la difficulté d'obtenir en fin d'expérimentation le complexe totalement privé de phase aqueuse.

Filtration sur gel

Principe de la filtration sur gel (Determan, 1968)   La filtration sur gel de dextran (Séphadex) tend de plus en plus à remplacer la dialyse en raison de sa rapidité d'exécution.

Les macromolécules de dextran forment un réseau tridimensionnel de chaînes polysaccharidiques permettant une séparation des molécules dans l'ordre décroissant de leurs masses moléculaires. Dans un tel système, les molécules dont les dimensions sont supérieures aux plus gros pores du gel gonflé traversent directement le gel dans la phase liquide interne et seront éluées les premières ('principe d'exclusion'); par contre, les petites molécules diffuseront en fonction de leur taille et de leur forme dans la phase liquide interne du gel et seront éluées ultérieurement. Par une telle technique on pourra séparer le complexe macromoléculaire (PT) de l'excès du toxique. Pour cela il conviendra de choisir un réseau dont le domaine de fractionnement en poids moléculaire interdisant aux macromolécules de type (PT) de diffuser dans la phase aqueuse interne du gel, possibilité seule réservée aux petites molécules du toxique.

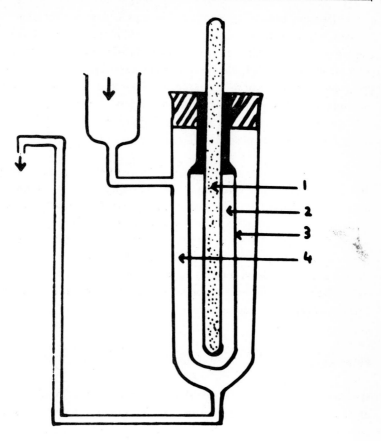

FIGURE 10.   Dialyse dynamique Schéma d'aprés Vo Phi Hung (1966)
1) baguette de verre
2) compartiment interne
3) membrane semi perméable
4) compartiment externe

Technique originelle d'etude (Wilcox et Lisowski, 1960; Ekman et al., 1961; De Moor et al., 1962; Acred et al., 1963; Batchelor et al., 1967; Determan, 1968) Si placés dans ces conditions optimales quant au choix de la matrice nous en éluons un milieu réactionnel contenant le complexe (PT) et l'excès d'ion toxique en dosant dans chaque fraction la protéine et le toxique, nous aurons un diagramme d'élution présentant 2 pics: le premier maximum correspondant au complexe, le deuxième à la fraction toxique libre (graphique no. 11). Généralement on définit la position des pics par leur K_D (co-

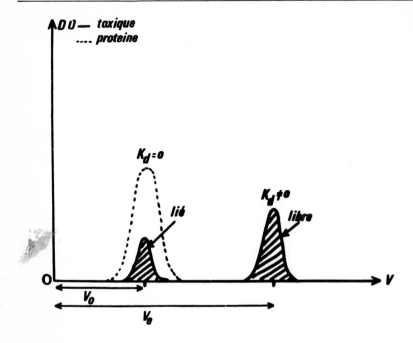

FIGURE 11.   Séparation du complexe protéine toxique, de la fraction libre du toxique par filtration sur gel de Séphadex, diagramme d'élution

efficient de partage de la molécule considérée entre la phase aqueuse externe du grain de gel et sa phase aqueuse interne). Cette valeur est calculée à partir de la relation

$$K_D = \frac{V_e - V_s}{V_i}$$

V_o représente le volume de la phase aqueuse externe du gel; il est égal au volume d'élution d'une substance dont le p.m. interdit sa diffusion à l'intérieur du gel. Donc, pour une telle substance, on aura $K_D = 0$; c'est le cas du complexe (PT).

V_i représente le volume de la phase aqueuse interne du gel. Il est égal à:

$$V_i = V_t - V_o - m_g V_g$$

V_t est le volume total de la colonne de gel utilisé, m_g le poids de gel mis en oeuvre, V_g le volume spécifique de la matrice ($V_g \simeq 0,6$)

V_o représente le volume d'élution de (PT) ou (P).

De ces considérations il ressort que le complexe (PT) aura un K_D égal à 0, alors que le K_D du toxique sera supérieur à 0. Généralement, il est préférable d'utiliser un Séphadex G25 dont la limite d'exclusion en poids moléculaire est de 5,000, les petites molécules ayant généralement dans ces conditions un K_D compris entre 0,8 et 1 (Barlow *et al.*, 1962).

De nombreux travaux ont été consacrés à l'étude comparative des résultats obtenus par dialyse et sur Séphadex. De ces etudes il apparaît une possibilité d'erreur pour la filtration sur gel (Ekman *et al.*, 1961; Remenant, 1966; Vo Phi Hung, 1966); certains complexes (PT) pouvant être retransfomés en leurs composants P et T par une réaction du type

$$P - T + gel \rightleftharpoons P + gel - T$$

Pour pallier cette difficulté, Wilcox et coll. (1960) ont utilisé comme éluant, dans le cas précis de l'étude de la fixation des métaux, des tampons au formiate d'ammonium. La technique de Hummel et Dreyer apporte la solution la plus heureuse à cette difficulté car son utilisation peut être généralisée.

Technique modifiée de Hummel par Dreyer (1962) La solution de la substance chimique étudiée (T) sert d'une part à constituer le gel du support et d'autre part à l'élution du complexe. La manipulation est réalisée en une seule opération. Après application de l'échantillon de solution de contact, l'analyse spectrophotométrique de (T) dans l'effluant permet de repérer:

1) un pic positif correspondant au complexe (P.T.) tranchant sur la ligne de base correspondant à la concentration moyenne du toxique dans l'effluant;

2) un pic négatif correspondant au volume de rétention de la substance (voir graphique no. 12).

Cette technique nous paraît satisfaisante car elle évite la dissociation éventuelle du complexe (PT).

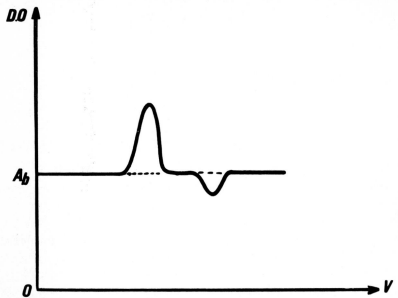

FIGURE 12.   Diagramme d'élution obtenu par la méthode de Hummel et Dreyer
Ab = absorption de référence (ligne de base)

Ultérieurement, Fairclough et Fruton (1966) ont précisé la valeur pratique
de cette méthode en comparant d'une part leurs résultats expérimentaux à
ceux obtenus par dialyse et en donnant d'autre part une formule corrective de
la valeur de la fraction fixée par estimation de l'aire du pic négatif. Si dans les
'i' fractions correspondant à ce pic nous avons pour chacune d'elle un abaisse-
ment Δ A_i de la densité optique par rapport à la ligne de base (Ab), le
nombre de micromoles fixés sera:

$$F = \frac{\Sigma_i \left(\Delta A_i . V_i \right)}{\mu \, \text{mole} \in \times \, 10^{-3}}$$

où $\in$ est le coefficient d'extinction molaire de (T) et V_i le volume de chaque
fraction d'élution en millilitres.

La valeur de F doit être corrigée en tenant compte de la dilution apportée
lors de l'application sur la colonne de la solution aqueuse de protéine par la
soustraction de la quantité: 'f' égale à:

$$f = \frac{\left[A_b \; P \quad W - V\,(1-W)\right]}{\in}$$

Dans cette égalité:

A_b représente la densité optique de la ligne de base

P la quantité de protéine (mg)

W la teneur en eau de l'échantillon protéique exprimée en fraction décimale

V volume spécifique partiel de la protéine (pour le sérum albumine 0,74 ml/g.)

Avantage de la filtration sur gel Outre la rapidité des techniques proposées (Kakei et Glass, 1962; Acred *et al.*, 1963) qui permettent la réalisation dans certains cas d'analyses cliniques de routine (De Moor *et al.*, 1962; Barber *et al.*, 1963), un des avantages de la méthode et de la variante de Hummel et Dreyer réside en la détermination possible du poids moléculaire du complexe (P.T.) formé. Pour cela, il suffit de choisir un support dont les caractéristiques permettent un partage entre les deux phases du gel du complexe (P.T.) isolé au cours des précédentes opérations (Hardy et Mansford, 1962). Il y a une relation quasi linéaire entre le logarithme des poids moléculaires d'une part et le volume d'élution d'autre part (Acred *et al.*, 1963; Whitaker, 1963; Leach et O'Shea, 1965). Expérimentalement, il suffira conc d'étalonner au préalable la colonne à l'aide de quelques protéines de poids moléculaire connu pour déterminer en fonction du volume d'élution le poids moléculaire du complexe. La connaissance de ce poids moléculaire peut dans certains cas se révéler très précieuse et permettre la mise en évidence de dimérisation ou de polymérisation des protéines.

Parmi les autres possibilités expérimentales qu'offrent ces méthodes il convient de mentionner la détermination des principaux paramètres thermodynamiques de la réaction dont entre autres, la variation d'énergie libre standard Δ F, ainsi que la variation d'enthalpie standard Δ H. Pour cela il suffira de déterminer classiquement la constante K à plusieurs températures et d'exploiter graphiquement ces résultats.

En toxicologie, la mise en évidence de compétitions entre deux substances en vue de l'occupation d'un site est parfois fondamentale pour l'interprétation d'un mode d'action toxique. Les techniques qui viennent d'être décrites se prêtent bien souvent à une telle démonstration, à condition que les deux substances étudiées simultanément aient des volumes d'élution différents (Fairclough et Fruton, 1966).

MATERIEL EXPERIMENTAL

Après l'exposé des techniques utilisables pour déterminer la réactivité des substances chimiques à l'égard des protéines sériques, il y a lieu d'envisager les critéres qui peuvent guider l'expérimentation dans le choix:
—du matériel protéique,
—des substances chimiques à tester,
—des milieux réactionnels.

Choix du materiel proteique

Le matériel protéique utilisé dans l'étude expérimentale de la fixation devra être choisi en fonction des données toxicologiques et pharmacologiques. Cependant le plus souvent il est primordial de localiser tout d'abord l'impact sanguin de la substance étudiée; pour cela, les globules rouges (suspension lavée) et les protéines sériques peuvent être étudiées séparément. Ce premier travail peut être complété judicieusement par un examen du comportement des éléments protéiques fractionnés car il est facile d'obtenir soit commercialement, soit au laboratoire, les différentes fractions plasmatiques de Cohn (graphique no. 13).

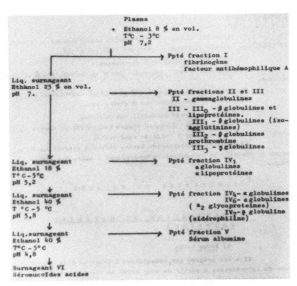

FIGURE 13   Fractionnement des protéines plasmatiques par la méthode de cohn

Cette étude devra refléter quantitativement la composition normale des protéines mises en oeuvre afin de révéler une affinité particulière par simple comparaison avec le mélange initialement testé. Parmi les protéines sériques l'albumine se révèle souvent comme la plus réactive (Brodie et Hogben, 1957; Stafford, 1962a et b). Par exemple, dans le cas des crésols (graphique no. 1) sa contribution au phénomène global est de plus de 80% (Fauran, 1968, 1969).

A côté de la détermination des éléments contribuant à révéler l'impact sanguin du toxique, il est tout aussi important de définir le comportement des éléments protéiques cellulaires et plus particulièrement, compte tenu de leur rôle biochimique, celui des acides nucléiques. A cet égard les interactions peuvent se révéler par l'inhibition de certains processus biosynthétiques d'importance primordiale. Par exemple les dérivés de l'actinomycine, de la chromomycine, de l'acridine ainsi que les anthracyclines, en se fixant fortement sur l'hélice de l'ADN, inhiberont la RNA polymérase DNA dépendante et des lors, la synthèse des ARN.

Il est parfois possible de préciser le mécanisme de la fixation en s'adressant à plusieurs types d'acides nucléiques différents par leur composition en base azotée. Dans le cas des ADN, on pourra très facilement faire varier la concentration en guanine et cytosine (G + C) en utilisant par exemple les ADN de:

Cytophaga johnsonii	(G + C = 34%)	
Bacillus subtilis	(G + C = 43%)	
Escherichia coli B	(G + C = 50%)	d'après Kersten *et al.* (1966).
Sarcina lutea	(G + C = 71%)	

Parmi les autres possibilités techniques qui peuvent se révéler fécondes en enseignements susceptibles de préciser les modalités chimiques de la fixation, nous signalerons l'utilisation d'agents de dénaturation des protéines agissant par des mécanismes définis (Kautzmann, 1959). Pour les protéines sériques, l'urée est particulièrement utilisée (Teresi et Luck, 1948; Fauran *et al.*, 1967b; Fauran, 1968). Dans le cas des acides nucléiques, c'est la modification des profils des courbes de dénaturation thermique en fonction de la densité optique qui sera particulièrement intéressante (Kersten *et al.*, 1966).

Choix des substances chimiques etudiees

Le nombre des substances médicamenteuses et toxiques est impressionnant aujourd'hui comme en témoignent les revues réalisées en 1949 par Goldstein et en 1965 par Truhaut (Truhaut, 1965).

A côté des critères de pureté des substances chimiques testées que l'on étudie il est parfois souhaitable de pouvoir disposer de molécules de structure voisine afin de déterminer les éléments structuraux conditionnant leur réactivité à l'égard du matériel protéique. Pour cela il y a tout lieu de s'adresser à des séries chimiques homogènes pour lesquelles on disposera de données physico-chimiques précises. En effet il est par exemple important de connaître la constante de dissociation des éléments d'une série homologue; c'est ainsi que, suivant que la fixation évolue dans le même sens ou en sens contraire de la dissociation ionique, une liaison de type salin pourra ou non être envisagée (voir graphique no. 14). Bien d'autres paramètres physiques

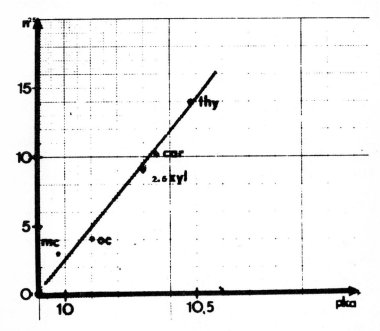

FIGURE 14.   Etude de la fixation de certains crésols en lonction de leur pK_a d'aprés Fauran (1968)

mc = méta−crésol
oc = ortho−crésol
2−5 xyl = 2−5−xylénol
car = carvacrol
thy = thymol

Le nombre de molécules fixées par mole de protéine évoluant dans le même sens que le pK_a on peut dire que plus le phénol sera dissocié en ses ions, moins il se fixera. Dès lors une liaison saline entre la protéine et le phénol est peu probable.

peuvent contribuer à définir les éléments structuraux conditionnant la fixation, notamment l'encombrement stérique et le coefficient de partage entre
une phase polaire ou apolaire (Caujolle *et al.*, 1968).

Choix du milieu reactionnel   Afin de se placer dans des conditions expérimentales aussi voisines que possible de la réalité physiologique, le choix
rigoureux du pH du milieu réactionnel s'impose. Pour la fixation sur les
protéines sériques on retient le plus souvent le sérum physiologique ou des
solutions tampons de pH 7.35–7.40. Il est important en outre de préciser la
force ionique des solutions tampons; il semble logique de déterminer celle-ci
de façon à ce qu'elle corresponde à l'osmolarité du sérum physiologique (300
milliosmoles). Dans nos expériences nous utilisons un tampon phosphate de
pH 7.60, de molarité 0.2, ce qui correspond à une osmolarité très voisine de
300 milliosmoles. Pour les expérimentations conduites par filtration sur gel,
cette force ionique est en outre suffisante pour éviter tout phénomène
parasite.

Il est parfois nécessaire de faire une étude à différents pH: Chambon *et
al.* (1968) ont pu montrer que l'amodiaquine et la chloroquine se fixent
beaucoup plus sur les protéines à des pH supérieurs au pH physiologique,
alors que la fixation est plus faible, pour des valeurs de pH inférieures. Dans le
cas de la chloroquine, l'élimination urinaire évolue de façon analogue.

CONCLUSION

L'étude de la fixation sur les macromolécules protéiques des poisons et des
médicaments est susceptible de trouver des applications d'un très grand
intérêt dans les domaines toxicologique, thérapeutique, immunologique et
biochimique.

Ce phénomène n'est pas seulement une 'adsorption,' au sens physique de
ce terme.

Le point capital des recherches à entreprendre réside dans la détermination
des modalités de l'action quelquefois réversible de la substance sur la
protéine, cause première de diverses manifestations biochimiques décelables
par des techniques appropriées.

Compte tenu de nos propres expériences, les méthodes analytiques choisies
ne peuvent être satisfaisantes que moyennant une définition rigoureuse des
paramètres structuraux et thermodynamiques de la réaction protéine-
substance chimique.

Plusieurs types de liaison peuvent être contractés simultanément entre le poison ou le médicament d'une part et la protéine d'autre part: à côté des liaisons classiquement définies (ioniques, covalentes) ou des liaisons hydrogènes, il convient bien souvent d'examiner aussi, pour la combinaison protéine-substance chimique, la possibilité de liaisons improprement considérées comme secondaires soit par des forces du type Van der Waals, soit par polarité hydrophobe soit encore par transfert de charge.

Nous nous proposons de définir dans un prochain travail différentes modalités de combinaisons protéine-substance chimique.

Bibliographie

Acred, P., D. M. Brown, T. L. Hardy et K. R. L. Mansford 1963 'A new approach to studying the protein-binding properties of penicillins.' *Nature*, 199: 758−759.

Andrews, P. 1964 'Estimation of the molecular weights of proteins by Sephadex gel-filtration.' *J. Biochem.*, 91: 222−233.

Barber, A. A., C. Dempster et N. G. Anderson 1963 'A gel filtration method for studies on protein-iron binding.' *Clin. Chim. Acta*, 8: 143−145.

Barlow, C. F., H. Firemark et L. J. Roth 1962 'Drug-plasma binding measured by Sephadex.' *J. Pharm. Pharmacol.*, 14: 550−555.

Batchelor, F. R., J. G. Feinberg, J. M. Dewdney and R. D. Weston 1967 'A penicilloylated protein impurity as a source of allergy to benzylpenicillin and 6-aminopenicillanic acid.' *Lancet*, 1: 1175−1177.

Beaven, G. H. et E. R. Holiday 1952 'Ultraviolet absorption spectra of proteins and amino acids.' *In*: Anson, M. L. (ed.), *Advances in Protein Chemisty*, 7: 319−386. Academic Press, New York.

Brodie, B. B. et C. A. M. Hogben 1957 'Some physico-chemical factors in drug action.' *J. Pharm. Pharmacol.*, 9: 345−380.

Caujolle, F., F. Fauran et Dang Quoc Quan 1968 'Sur la liaison entre la sérum albumine bovine et les métacrèsols 6 monoalkylés.' *Compt. Rend. Acad. Sci.*, 267: 2213−2215.

Chambon, P., Vo Phi Hung et J. M. Remenant 1968 'Enquête expérimentale sur le métabolisme de quelques médicaments antimalariques: chloroquine et amodiaquine. Bordeaux Médical.' 8: 1471−1477.

De Moor P., K. Heirwegh, J. F. Heremans et M. Declerck-Raskin 1962 'Protein binding of corticoids studied by gel filtration.' *J. Clin. Invest.*, 41: 816−827.

Determan, H. 1968 '*Gel Chromatography.*' Springer-Verlag, New York.

Duggan, E. L. et J. M. Luck 1948 'The combination of organic anions with serum albumin. IV. Stabilization against urea denaturation.' *J. Biol. Chem.*, **172**: 205–220.

Eichhorn, G. L., P. Clark et E. D. Becker 1966 'Interactions of Metal ions with Polynucleotides and related compounds. VII. The binding of copper II to nucleosides, nucleotides and deoxyribonucleic acids.' *Biochemistry*, **5**: 245–252.

Ekman, L., E. Valmet et B. Aberg 1961 'Behavior of yttrium –91 and some lanthanons towards serum proteins in paper electrophoresis, density gradient electrophoresis and gel filtration.' *Intern. J. Appl. Radiation Isoto.*, **12**: 32–41.

Fairclough, G. F., Jr. et J. S. Fruton 1966 'Peptide-protein interaction as studied by gel filtration.' *Biochemistry*, **5**: 673–683.

Fauran, F., A. Alvinerie et M. Bonnafous 1967a 'Fixation des crésols es des méthylisopropyl phénols sur les protéines sériques bovines.' Assemblée générale de l'union médicale de la Méditerranée Latine. *Symposium de Toxicologie experimentale*, Toulouse.

Fauran, F., M. Bonnafous et A. Alvinerie 1967b 'Fixation *in vitro* des phénols substitués sur les fractions albuminiques et globuliniques bovines.' *Toulouse Pharm.*, **14**: 119–123.

Fauran, F. 1968 'Contribution a l'Etude de la Fixation Proteinique et du Metabolisme des o et m Cresols.' Thèse Doct. Etat Pharm. Toulouse, no. 34.

Fauran, F. 1969 'Rôle de l'encombrement stérique dans la fixation des méta-crésols ortho alkylés sur la sérum albumine bovine.' *VIemes Journees Medicales de Dakar*.

Goldstein, A. 1949 'The interaction of drugs and plasma proteins.' *Pharmacol. Rev.*, **1**: 102–165.

Hardy, T. L. et K. R. L. Mansford 1962 'Gel filtration as a method of studying drug-protein binding.' *J. Biochem.*, **83**: 34–35.

Hugues, T. R. et I. M. Klotz 1960 'Analysis of metal protein complexes.' *In*: Glick, D. (ed.), *Methods of Biochemical Analysis*. Vol. 3, pp. 265–299. Interscience, New York.

Hummel, J. P. et W. J. Dreyer 1962 'Measurement of protein-binding phenomena by gel filtration.' *Biochim. Biophys. Acta*, **63**: 530–532.

Kakei, M. et G. B. J. Glass 1962 'Separation of bound and free Vit B_{12} on Sephadex G-25 column.' *Proc. Soc. Exp. Biol. Med.*, **3**: 270–271.

Kautzmann, W. 1959 'Some factors in the interpretation of protein denaturation.' *In*: Anfinsen, C. B., Jr., M. L. Anson, K. Bailey and J. T. Edsall (eds.), *Advances in Protein Chemistry*, **19**: 1–63. Academic Press, New York.

Kersten, W., H. Kersten, W. Szybalski et M. Fiandt 1966 'Physiocochemical properties of complexes between Deoxyribonucleic acid and Antibiotics which affect ribonucleic acid synthesis.' *Biochemistry*, **5**: 236–244.

Koshland, D. E., G. Nemety et D. Filmer 1966 'Comparison of experimental binding data and theoretical models in proteins containing subunits.' *Biochemistry*, **5**: 365–385.

Leach, A. A. et P. C. O'Shea 1965 'The determination of up to 225,000 by gel filtration on a single column of Sephadex G-200 at 25° and 40°.' *J. Chromatog.*, **17**: 245–251.

Löber, G. 1964 'Mesures de la fluorescence effectuées sur des complexes de colorant et du DNA à l'aide du monochromateur à miroirs SPM2.' *Revue d'Iena*.

Meunier, M. T. 1961 '*Contribution a l'Etude de la Liaison de quelques Medicaments aux Proteines Seriques*.' Thèse Doct. Univ. Pharm. Clermont-Ferrand, no. 3.

Monod, J., J. P. Changeux et F. Jacob 1963 'Allosteric proteins and cellular control systems.' *J. Mol. Biol.*, 6: 306–329.

Remenant, J. M. 1966 *'Contribution a l'Etude Toxicologique du Metabolisme et de l'Elimination de l'Amodiaquine.'* Thèse Doct. Etat Pharm., Lyon, no. 29.

Salvatore, G., M. Andreolli et J. Roche 1966 'Thyroid hormones-plasma interaction.' *In*: Degrex, P. et P. M. de Traverse (eds.), *West European Symposium on Clinical Chemistry, Proceedings of the Symposium on the Transport Function of Plasma Proteins*. Elsevier, Amsterdam, 5.

Scatchard, G. 1949 'The attractions of proteins for small molecules and ions.' *Ann. N.Y. Acad. Sci.*, 51: 660–672.

Scatchard, G. et E. S. Black 1949 *'J. Phys. Colloid Chem.,'* 53: 88. Cité par Hugues et Klotz (1960).

Seegers, W. H. 1943 'A convenient arrangement for rapid dialysis.' *J. Lab. Clin. Med.*, 28: 897–898.

Stafford, W. L. 1962a 'The binding by bovine plasma and plasma fractions of salicylic acids and some of its 3. Alkyl analogues.' *Biochem. Pharmacol.*, 11: 685–692.

Stafford, W. L. 1962b 'Protein binding of salicylates.' *'Salicylates' Int. Symposium.*

Teresi, J. D. et J. M. Luck 1948 'The combination of organic anions with serum albumin. VI. Quantitative studies by equilibrium dialysis.' *J. Biol. Chem.*, 174: 653–661.

Thorp, J. M. 1964 'The influence of plasma proteins on the action of drugs.' *In*: *Absorption and Distribution of Drugs*. pp. 64–76. Livingstone, Edimburg-London.

Truhaut, R. 1966 'The transportation of toxic compounds by plasma proteins.' *In*: Degrex, P. et P. M. de Traverse (eds.), *West European Symposium on Clinical chemistry. Proceedings of the Symposium on the transport function of plasma proteins*. Elsevier, Amsterdam, 5: 147–171.

Vo Phi Hung 1966 *'Etude du Metabolisme et de l'Elimination de la Chloroquine.'* These Doct. Etat Pharm., Lyon, no. 24.

Whitaker, J. R. 1963 'Determination of molecular weights of proteins by gel filtration on Sephadex.' *Anal. Chem.*, 35: 1950–1953.

Wilcox, P. E. et J. Lisowski 1960 'Applications of gel filtration in studies of protein-metal complexes.' *Federation Proc.*, 19: 333.